# The ART
## *of*
# FINGER WAVING

*By* PAUL COMPAN

Copyright © 2007 by Bramcost Publications
All rights reserved
Published in the United States of America

This Bramcost Publications edition is an unabridged republication of the rare original work.

www.BramcostPublications.com

ISBN 10: 1-934268-34-8
ISBN 13: 978-1-934268-34-6

Library of Congress Control Number: 2008926256

Bramcost Publications

# INDEX TO LESSONS

## PART ONE
*Fundamental Principles in Finger Waving Technique*

| | | |
|---|---|---:|
| I. | Definition of Finger Waving. | |
| | Preparing the Hair for Waving. | |
| | Curling Fluids | 7 |
| II. | Technique of the Movement | 9 |
| III. | Matching Waves (Horse-Shoe Waving) | 13 |

## PART TWO
*The Three General Types of Swirl Waves*

| | | |
|---|---|---:|
| IV. | Swirl No. 1 | 15 |
| V. | Swirl No. 2 | 17 |
| VI. | Swirl No. 3 | 18 |

## PART THREE
*Popular Finger-Waved Hair Styles*

| | | |
|---|---|---:|
| VII. | Pompadour Finger Waving | 20 |
| VIII. | The Varsity Bob | 23 |
| IX | The French Cocktail Bob | 26 |
| X. | The Lorelei Bob | 30 |
| XI. | The Windblown Bob | 32 |
| XII. | The Extreme French Swirl | 35 |
| XIII. | The "Whoopee" Bob | 37 |
| XIV. | The Cincy Bob | 41 |
| XV. | The Long Bob | 45 |
| XVI. | The Billie Dove Bob | 48 |
| XVII. | The Clara Bow Bob | 51 |
| XVIII. | The "Push-Up" Wave | 55 |

# FOREWORD

FINGER WAVING is possibly the newest branch of beauty culture, yet in its few years of existence it has reached an importance that few phases of the art enjoy. Very little has been written on the subject, and there is a great demand for instructive literature on finger waving being made throughout the country, not only by those just entering the profession, but also by hairdressers whose training preceded the era of finger waving and who want to add this profitable art to their beauty culture knowledge.

In the preparation of this book the point of view of both the student and the experienced hairdresser has been considered. Observations of the author have led him to believe that the training needed for the experienced beauty culturist is practically the same as that required by the beginning student, because of the vast differences between finger waving and any other beauty culture practice; for that reason the fundamental principles in the technique of finger waving have been brought out emphatically in the opening lessons. General styles adaptable to the average shapes of heads are explained in detail and illustrated with actual photographs, as well as many individual hair styles designed for the many different types of beauty.

Never before, however, has an analysis of the actual individual movements in the technique of the wave been explained and illustrated as has been attempted in this treatise on finger waving.

Many practicable styles of coiffures, both for short hair and long, are shown and explained in this book as well. Some of the individual styles have appeared in various numbers of MODERN BEAUTY SHOP Magazine, and they are reprinted herewith to provide a complete study. These styles have been selected with great care and it is hoped that the student of finger waving will find them an exceptionally helpful and profitable study indeed.

M. H. C.

# The Art of Finger Waving

## LESSON I

### DEFINITION OF FINGER WAVING
### PREPARING THE HAIR FOR WAVING
### CURLING FLUIDS

FINGER WAVING is the shaping or moulding of the hair while wet into "s"-curved undulations with the fingers and comb. These waves when dried without being disturbed will fall into beautiful deep waves. Finger waving differs from marcel waving in that there are no irons used on the hair. Not only naturally curly or permanently waved hair can be finger waved, but it is equally successful on straight hair.

In preparing the hair for finger waving, the first requisite, of course, is that the hair is clean. Finger waving can be done especially well after a shampoo inasmuch as the hair must be wet to insert the wave. Some hairdressers prefer to dry the hair after it has been washed before wetting it again for the finger wave (on the same principle that clothes are allowed to dry thoroughly before they are dampened for ironing). Most patrons prefer, however, to have a finger wave immediately follow the shampoo, and in most beauty shops the time element is so valuable that it is a far more practicable procedure.

After being washed, the hair must be thoroughly dampened with water or curling fluid and combed completely free of all snarls whatsoever. If the hair is naturally wavy or if the patron has been given a perfect permanent wave, the finger wave can be inserted when the hair has been wet with water only.

A word about curling fluids: There are numerous types and numerous brands on the market, many of which are equally good. If the hair is clean, most curling fluids do not leave a flaky sediment on the hair and scalp. On oily hair, this sediment sometimes appears even though the hair has been thoroughly washed. In such cases the fluid should be more diluted and the hairdresser should brush this flakiness out of the hair before allowing the patron to leave the beauty shop.

The curling fluid should not be too thick when used on naturally curly hair or permanently waved hair. The hair will be much softer when dry if the wave has been inserted with curling fluid which has been diluted considerably with water. On straight hair which has no wave whatever in it, use the curling fluid or waving lotion without diluting it at all. As mentioned above, straight hair can be finger waved very successfully.

Nearly all manufacturers of waving lotions suggest their own methods of applying the curling fluid and have full directions on the bottle or on the package (if it is purchased in powdered form and diluted later). The procedure of applying curling fluid on straight hair is to rub the shaker containing the fluid all over the head, rubbing the fluid in well to soften the hair. Then take a towel and wipe off the excess lotion, leaving just enough on the hair so that it is thoroughly wet all over. This shortens the drying period.

It is a waste of time to apply the curling fluid with the comb. A shaker is very inexpensive and is more efficient to use and saves considerable time.

After applying the lotion, comb the hair through to the scalp until it is free of snarls, slanting always toward the back of the head. In combing the hair after the waving fluid has been applied, always start from the bottom of the hair, taking a small section at a time, working to the top of the head, to avoid creating the snarls which would occur if one started from the top or at the parting and combed down. In combing out a finger wave whether dry or wet remember to use this same method.

# THE ART OF FINGER WAVING

## LESSON II

### TECHNIQUE OF THE MOVEMENT

THERE are several primary steps in the actual execution of a finger wave and the technique of these movements must be thoroughly mastered by the finger waver before he or she attempts to wave a complete head. After much study and practice, a simplified outline of these individual movements has been arranged.

These are illustrated herewith, and it is suggested to the student that much attention be given to this lesson on technique as well as plenty of practice made before attempting to progress to the various styles illustrated and explained later in this book.

Comb the hair completely back and as smooth as possible after the hair has been dampened with the curling fluid. Use the

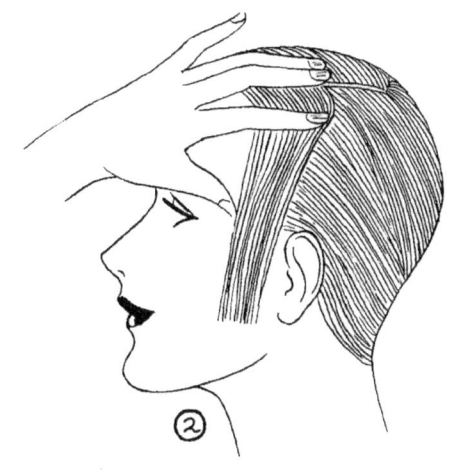

fine end of the comb to be sure that the hair is completely smooth and free of snarls, as in *Figure No.* 1 shown on the next page. Be sure to comb the hair clear through to the scalp. Many amateur finger wavers make the mistake of combing only the top layer of the hair. Consequently when the hair is dried and combed out it does not fall into regular deep waves, and the result of the effort is lost.

Next, place the forefinger about an inch or less from the parting, as shown in *Figure No.* 2. With the tip of the coarse side of the comb, take about an inch or an inch and one-half (in width) of the hair—through to the scalp—and comb it forward and down toward the face. *Figure No.* 3 illustrates

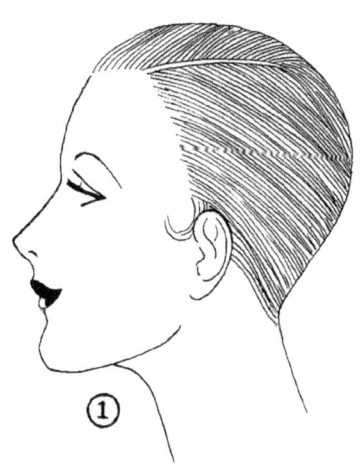

# THE ART OF FINGER WAVING

this movement. Press on the forefinger hard at the same time so that the hair which is turned back stays that way under the forefinger and does not turn forward.

Then take the hair which was turned forward, place the comb right next to the forefinger vertically and slide it about an inch or less. Be sure that it is not slid more than an inch because the wave will be too wide. Then, while holding the comb vertically, press on the forefinger well and roll the forefinger up and down against the comb to form the ridge of the wave, as is shown, too, in *Figure No. 3*.

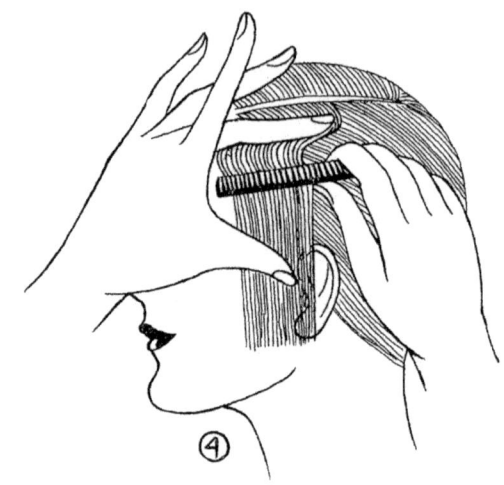

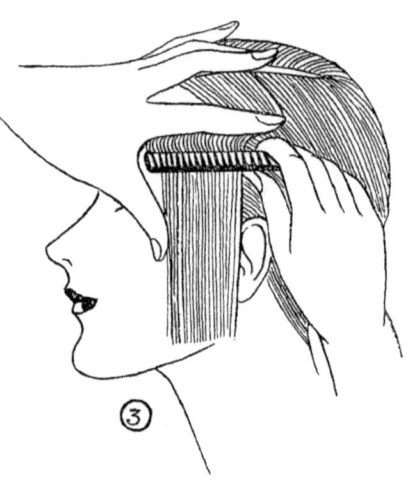

After forming the little ridge with the forefinger, place the second finger next to the comb where the forefinger was, as in *Figure No. 4*. Then flatten the comb and press the forefinger on it. Be sure that you don't press on the comb too hard with the forefinger because the more you press the more it scratches the customer's head. The proper position is shown in *Figure No. 5*.

After placing the forefinger on the comb,

slowly comb out the hair from underneath. Then press with both fingers, as illustrated also in *Figure No. 5*, holding the hair in position, making a ridge between the fingers. Then comb the hair all the way down to the ends.

Drop the forefinger a half inch below the ridge, but all the time make sure that the second finger is placed firmly and held firmly on the top of the ridge. Then press on the

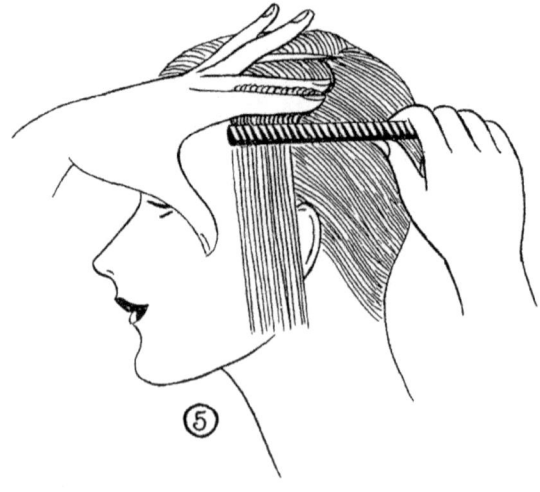

[ 10 ]

# THE ART OF FINGER WAVING

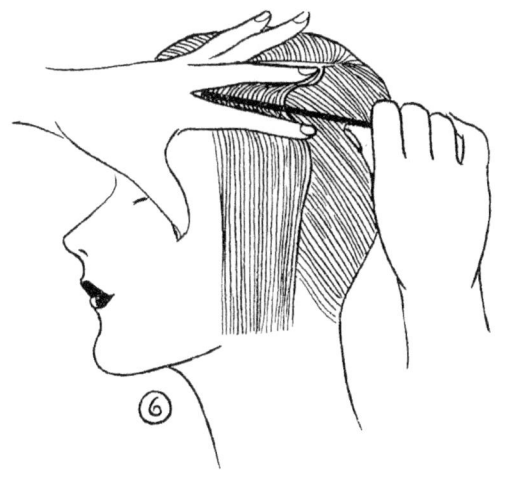

Get the ridge between the fingers again, slowly raise the comb to a vertical position and comb the wave out slowly as in *Figure No. 9*.

Then press and squeeze the ridge. Then repeat *Figures 6, 7, 8 and 9* until you obtain waves of the depth you desire.

Study the movements illustrated in the accompanying sketches carefully. Memorize the steps of the technique in their proper sequence and practice, practice, practice. Once the student masters these fundamental prin-

forefinger and press on the comb and raise the comb forward towards the second finger. This is shown in *Figure No. 6*.

Remove the comb; press with both fingers and squeeze the ridge as in *Figure No. 7*. To get a smooth and patent leather effect on the wave raise the forefinger straight up—press with the second finger; place the comb right next to the ridge and second finger and flatten it, as in *Figure No. 8*.

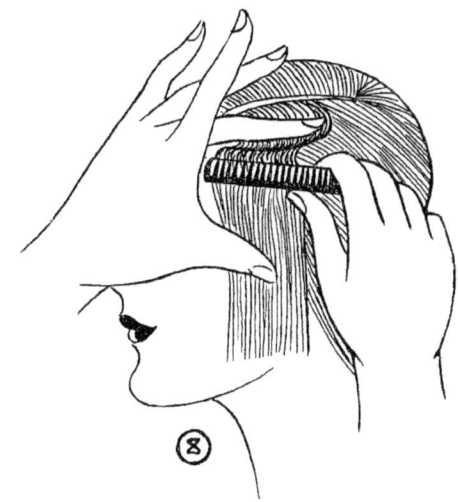

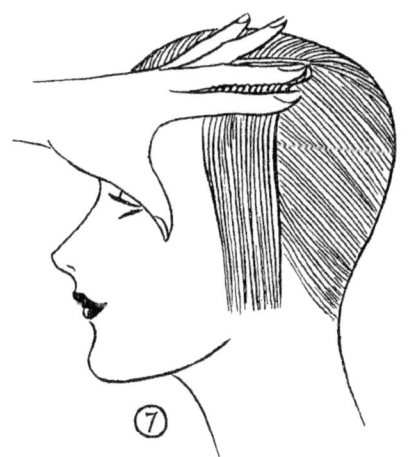

ciples, the secret of finger waving is his forever.

As a supplementary explanation, let us explain our term "ridge." Do not conflict this term with the sharp "railroad-track" edge of a marcel wave, commonly termed ridge also. For want of a better terminology for the lower and upper edges of the finger wave, these edges have been commonly called ridges and in this sense, a ridge is considered as artistic and in keeping with high-class

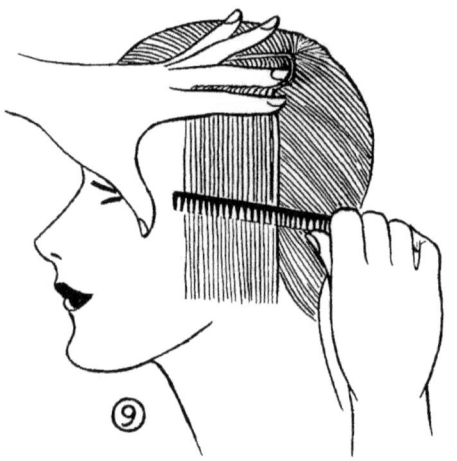

work as any other movement in the creating of a wave. In the following lessons the term will be used considerably so it is important that the student appreciate the sense in which it is applied.

If the patron insists that she does not want ridges in her waves just leave the waves as they are without raising the ridge but if a ridge is done properly, as illustrated in the sketches, when it is combed out it makes the wave look more natural and the waves stay in at least fifty per cent longer. You can turn to *Lesson* XVII to see how beautifully the "ridges" or edges of the waves appear when the hair is dry.

You will note by studying the photo mentioned that when the hair is dry the ridge is not at all stiff but merely an emphatic outline of the edge of the wave and lends an artistic sweep to the completed hairdress.

# LESSON III

## MATCHING WAVES
### (HORSE-SHOE WAVING)

IT IS OBVIOUS in finger waving that to get around a parting, either long or short, the waves would not match or blend into one another if one was started on each side and brought to the end of the parting. It is not correct to bring waves together in an inverted V-shape even around a long parting either. A circular effect must be obtained around the parting. To get this, one wave must be dropped close to the part to provide sufficient depth for the waves to

—or as they are sometimes called "half-waves." This is based on somewhat of the same principle as is used in marcel waving around partings when a horse-shoe effect is obtained in matching the waves.

The horse-shoe wave is used in matching waves around short partings or long partings. The short parting will be discussed first, and below are given two examples (1) a short parting horse-shoe wave with dips brought down low on the forehead and (2) a short

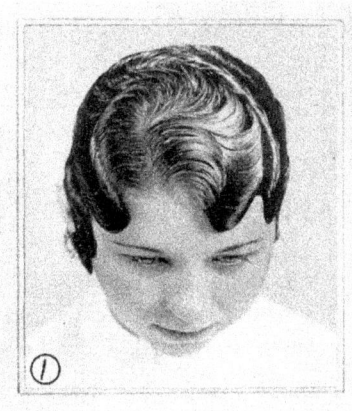 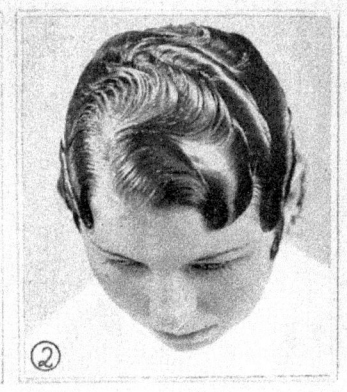

match properly around the parting. When thus perfectly matched the waves resemble the shape of a horseshoe, hence the name, "Horse-Shoe" wave.

Thus, in the proper matching of the waves, and also in the making of dips, occasionally it is necessary to lose or fade off short waves

parting horse-shoe wave in the "off-the-face" mode (more will be discussed later).

In fashioning either wave, comb the hair towards the back from the parting. Insert a wave on the heavy side of the hair and fade off toward the center. Note that the ridge of this wave is slanted diagonally toward the end of the parting in *Illustration No. 2*. It has a more circular sweep in that mode. In either case bring the second wave on the left (or heavy side) around the head, working it into the first wave on the right side and bringing the end of that wave out on the forehead into the dip. The style noted in *Illustration No. 2* can be worked off the ears if desired. This is not a popular fashion because a short-parting off-the-ear horse-shoe style has a tendency to add many years to a youthful person's appearance.

Short partings are not found very often, but in many cases where the back of the head is flat, the hair can be arranged to excellent advantage in this manner. Many times, too, a cowlick will prohibit a long parting and a desirable effect can be obtained with either of these short-parting horse-shoe fashions.

A beautiful and very popular "off-the-

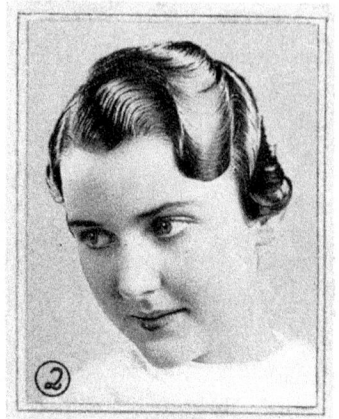

Figure 2a

face" style is shown in the long-parting horse-shoe mode pictured below. The first two waves—one on each side of the parting—are artistically tapered toward the parting and faded off and lost half-way to the end. This permits the hair to be swirled around the parting in a deep horse-shoe manner with the second wave on the right side being brought over to the left side, forming the first dip on that side just above the corner of the left eye. (*Illustration 1a.*) The side view of this fashion is shown in *Illustration 2a*.

In short bobs this mode is called the "Fifth Avenue" and the hair is brought slightly over the top of the ear and faded out to the shingle in the back. In long bobs or in long hair modes the hair is usually worn very low at the nape of the neck, either in closed turned-up curls or in a low close knot.

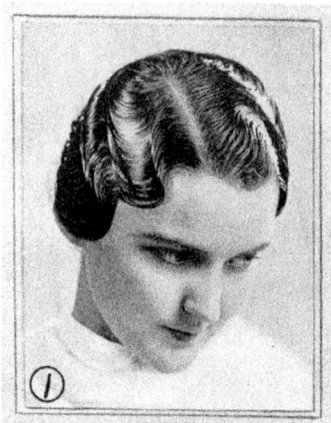

Figure 1a

# THE ART OF FINGER WAVING

## LESSON IV

### SWIRL NO. 1

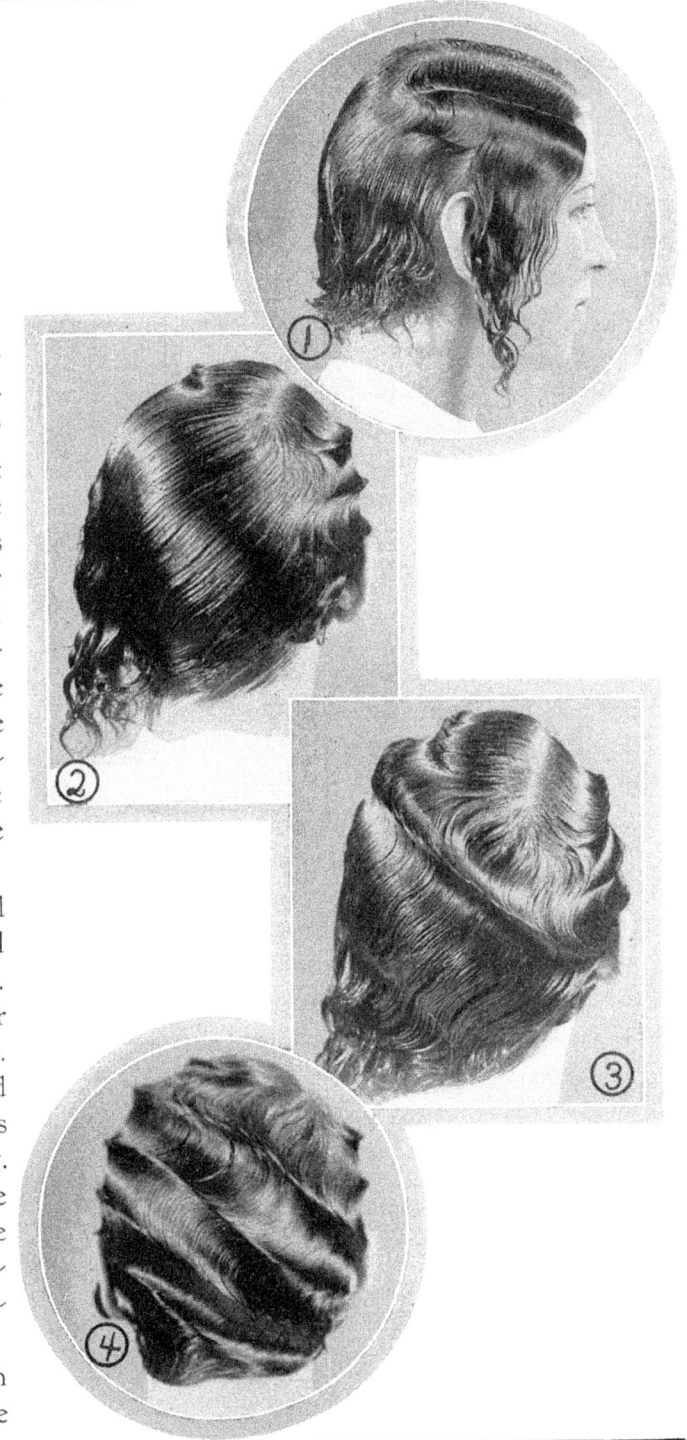

FINGER WAVING became universally popular with the introduction of the "Swirl Bob." Hairdressers quickly realized that novel and flattering effects could be achieved on various types of heads by digressing from the usual circular waves formerly so popular in marcel waving and artistically—not to mention easily—swirl the hair from one side gracefully to the other. The "Swirl Bob" became popular overnight and many hair artists owe their reputations to mastering the technique of this service.

There are three fundamental kinds of Swirl finger waves—Swirl No. 1, Swirl No. 2, and Swirl No. 3. These have been designed for the three general types of heads. Swirl No. 1 is suitable for the head in which the crown of the head is high on the same side as the parting.

Swirl No. 2 is used when the height of the crown is on one side (usually the heavy side of the parting) and the parting is on the opposite side.

Swirl No. 3 is the one in which the hair is extremely swirled all the way from one side over to the other. This is adaptable particularly to a head which is wide across and short from the crown to nape and neck. The parting can be on either the right or left side of the head.

We will explain and illustrate each of these fundamental swirl methods in the following lessons. If the student has mastered the technique of making a wave and the matching of the waves as explained in the previous pages, it will be only a matter of study and practice to learn the three types of swirl bobs and it will be comparatively simple to study and master the many styles shown in the following chapters.

Follow the simplified directions given below to execute this wave:

Comb and prepare the hair for finger waving as usual. Make your first ridge the proper length from the parting on the thin side of the hair (in this case illustrated the right side) usually one inch to one and one-half inches below. Work it all the way back to the end of the parting and start in where you left off to return toward the forehead with the second wave. *Illustration No. 1* shows the beginning of the second wave.

Complete the entire right side of the head in doing Swirl No. 1 before starting on the heavy side or, as in this case, the left side.

Comb the remaining hair toward the left side and insert the first ridge in the front of the head on the left side about one inch or one and one-half inches from the parting. Have it extended also to the length of the parting and gradually lose the wave, as shown in *Illustration No. 2*. In Swirl No. 1 it is necessary to bring third ridge from the right side diagonally across the crown of the head around into the second ridge on the left side, as shown in *Illustration No. 3*. Wave it all around from right side to the front of the head. This makes the first wave in the front or the left side.

When the wave is completed to the forehead, start back again bringing the third ridge on the left side around to the fourth ridge on the right side. In case the hair is too short for a fourth ridge on the front right side, fade off the ridge when it comes to the wave back of the ear. Complete the entire head, always working diagonally, as in *Illustration No. 4*.

In most cases this gives four deep waves and sometimes five in the back.

Turn up the ends of the hair on the left side in front toward the face (particularly for young women) or turn the ends back over the ear for those who demand such a coiffure.

# LESSON V

## SWIRL NO. 2

SWIRL NO. 2 differs from Swirl No. 1 in that the height of the crown of the head is on the opposite side of the parting and not on the same side as when Swirl No. 1 is used. The height of the crown can be on the left side and the parting on the right side or vice versa. In the pictures illustrated herewith, the height of the crown is on the left side and the parting on the right side.

Start finger waving the hair slightly closer to the parting than in Swirl No. 1. Put the first wave on the right side of the parting. Then start the first wave on the left side from the front. Come all the way around forming the ridge of this wave into the second ridge on the right side, as in *Illustration No. 1*. Note—the right side of the hair is *not* completely waved as down to the ends in Swirl No. 1. Each wave is done all the way around the head.

Make the third ridge on the right side and work from the front all the way around the head to the front of the left side forming the first deep wave on the left side.

Follow the waves all the way around the head in the same manner down to the ends diagonally across the head, as shown in *Illustration No. 2*. These usually result in about five deep waves in the back depending on how the hair is cut and the height of the head.

The ends of the hair can be finished off as in all swirl styles in upturned curls, sculptured curls, turned under or tapered as the hair will permit or the coiffure demands.

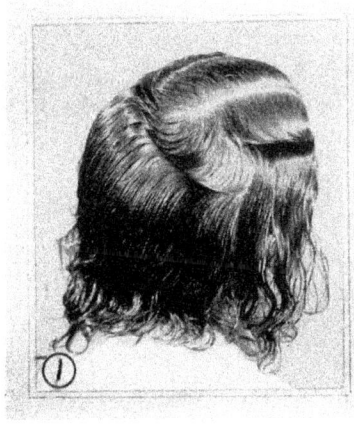
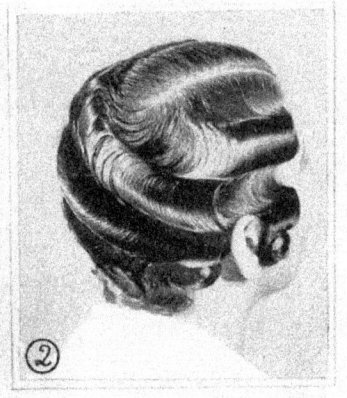

# THE ART OF FINGER WAVING

## LESSON VI

### SWIRL NO. 3

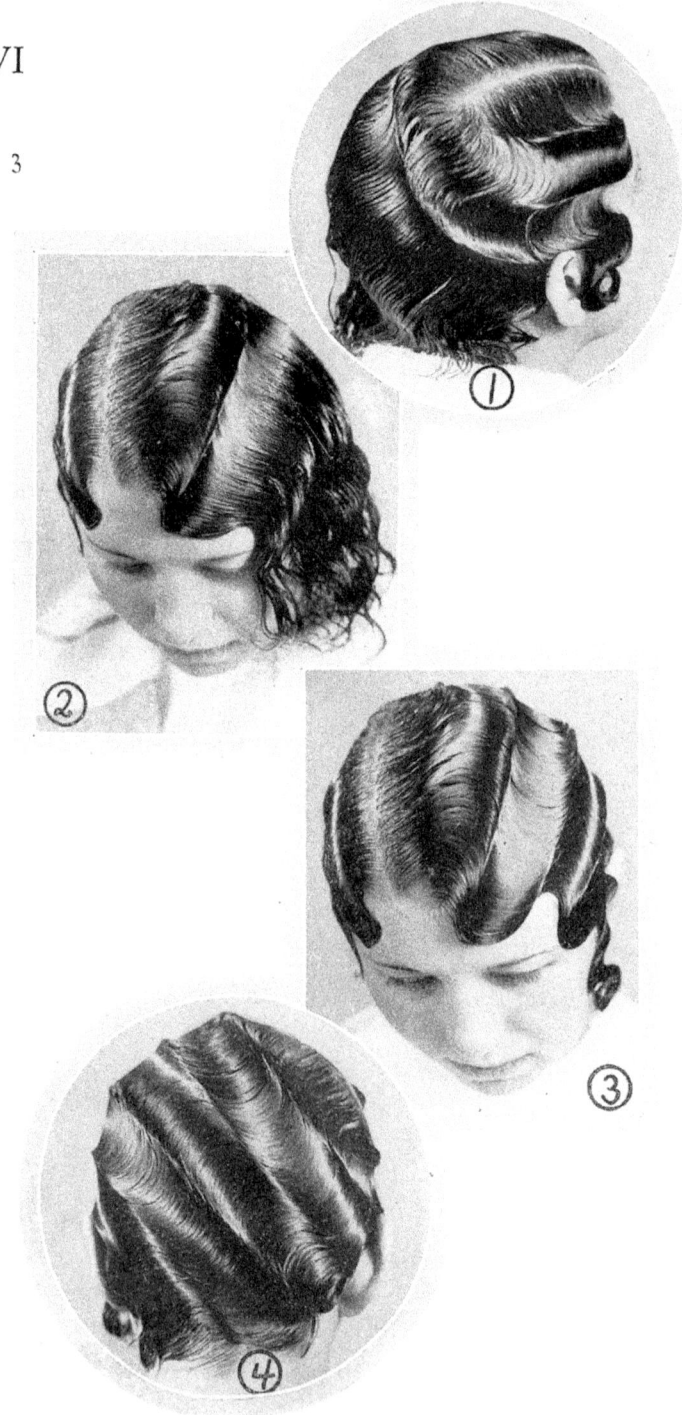

THIS extreme swirl is used on heads particularly short from the crown of the head to the nape of the neck but rather wide from ear to ear. Wave the right side down to the ends just as in *Illustration No. 1* of Swirl No. 1. Instead of working the second wave into the first on the left side, however, as done in Swirl No. 2, in Swirl No. 3 the third wave from the left side is brought over into the first wave on the right side.

*Illustration No.* 1 shows the completed right side and the way in which the third wave is worked around the head in an extreme swirl and brought over to the front on the left side.

An important feature in Swirl No. 3 is shown in *Illustration No. 2*. This is the fading out of the first ridge on the left side of the parting about in the middle of the parting. By fading out, we mean that the ridge gradually disappears so that the second ridge on the left side is brought down on the forehead and makes the first dip. This is an illustration of the matching

[ 18 ]

of the waves as was explained in *Lesson* III. The dip is brought low on the forehead, if the patron's features will permit, and the next ridge of that wave is formed and the wave is completed around the head and matched into the final right-side wave. Usually this wave is brought down to just behind the bottom of the ear and the next wave is started. It is shaped around the head and the second dip on the forehead on the left side falls just above the outside corner of the left eye as in *Illustration No. 3*. *Illustration No. 4* shows the four deep waves brought from the back directly to the front of the head on the left side and finished off on the left side over the ear —finishing the ends off in the style desired by the patron or fitting for her particular type.

# THE ART OF FINGER WAVING

## LESSON VII

### POMPADOUR FINGER WAVING

THE "OFF-THE-FACE" group of finger waving styles are perhaps the most difficult to master. There are many variations in this group and some are not as hard as others. The important factor to master here is when, how and where to "lose" the wave. As has been explained before, by losing a wave is

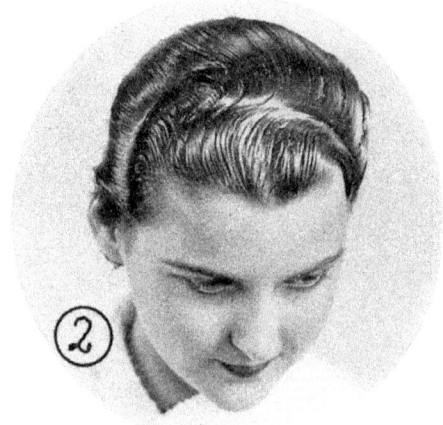

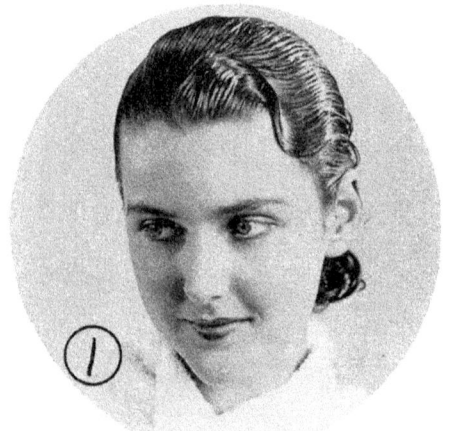

meant that the upper ridge of the wave is gradually tapered down and the hair is combed in the direction that the wave is being slanted until the end of the ridge actually fades off and disappears entirely and the remainder of that section of hair is blended off into the next wave.

Pompadours will be discussed particularly in this "off-the-face" group because the pompadour style is perhaps the most popular of this fashion. There are several kinds of pompadours—straight back with no dips, one dip, and two dips.

The straight back pompadour with no dips is illustrated below. The hair is combed straight back after it has been thoroughly dampened with curling fluid. Take a section of hair about half way across the forehead—insert the ridge of the first wave bringing the hair down in a straight slant to the left. Do

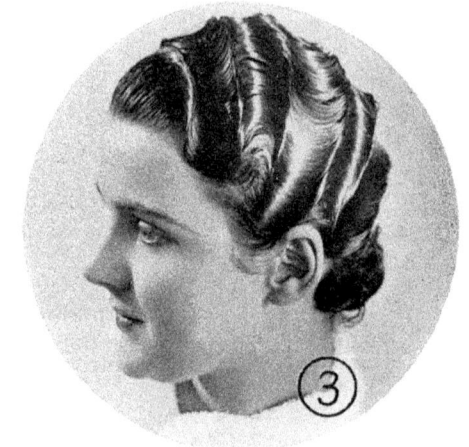

# THE ART OF FINGER WAVING

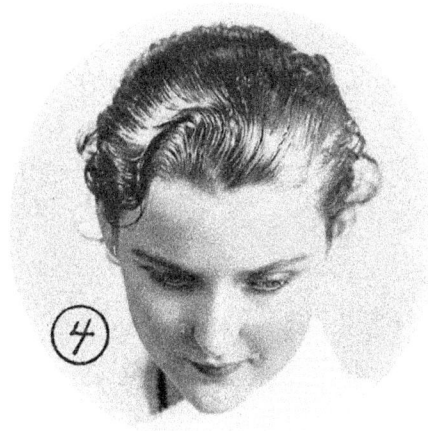

second ridge halfway completed. Finish finger waving the head in the same manner to the ends of the hair. In this fashion, which is usually worn by the mature matron rather than the younger woman, the hair is worn off the ears on both sides. Consequently take care not to bring the waves down very low on the sides of the head. *Illustration No.* 3 shows that the third wave extends only to the top of the ear, while the fourth wave ends just above the ear.

If the hair is long, the ends can be rolled into a graceful knot or arranged in a close-

not bring the hair out in a dip on the forehead in this wave. *Illustration No.* 1 shows the initial step in the no-dip pompadour.

Continue waving the first ridge of this wave, taking a small section of the hair at a time until the wave is completed to the right side. Start back from the right as always in finger waving, beginning where you left off and make the second wave. *Illustration No.* 2 shows the completed first ridge and the

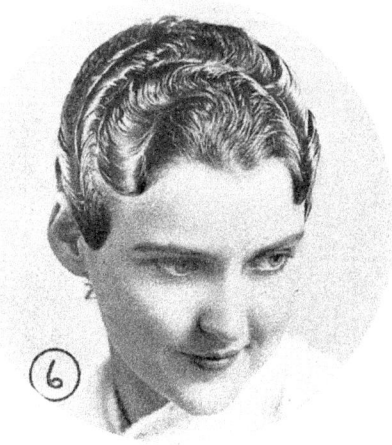

fitting figure 8 vertically or horizontally as the shape of the head permits. If the hair is short, a smart coiffure is arranged by shingling the hair just immediately above the normal hairline and having the final ridge of the last wave fade off into the shingle at the nape of the neck.

The pompadour with one or two dips is more complicated than the straight-back, off-the-ear type. It is necessary in this wave to lose the first ridge (from the right) at the center of the forehead. *Illustration No.* 5

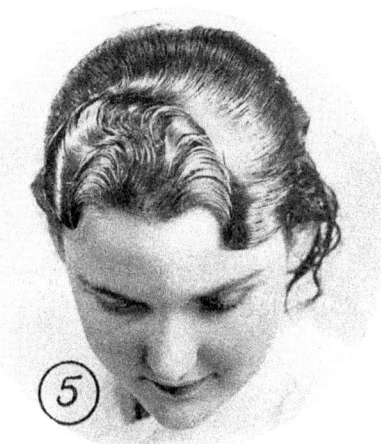

[ 21 ]

# THE ART OF FINGER WAVING

in this series shows the fading off of the first ridge just above the center of the forehead.

*Illustration No. 4* brings out in detail how this is accomplished. Take the section of hair on the right side of the head just above the corner of the eye. Insert the ridge of the first wave. Use the fine end of the comb to draw the hair into a dip out on the forehead. Continue inserting this first ridge as you work toward the center. Gradually lessen the ridge and fade off when the center is reached; combing the remainder of the hair in the direction you want the next wave to retain.

Comb the hair through the left side to be sure that the ridge is completely lost and start the first ridge on the left side by bringing the hair down with the fine end of the comb over the center of the left eye in the same manner as on the right side except that this dip is circled a little more than the first. The unevenness of these dips and the lack of studied exactness gives a decidedly artistic effect in the completed headdress.

*Illustration No. 6* shows how the third wave on the right side and the second wave on the left is brought out at least half-way down on the ear so that when the hair is dried the ears will be at least half covered. These dips can be brought down as low as the features will permit. The ends of the hair if short in the back can be fashioned into sculpture curls, tucked under, or, if sufficiently long, arranged in a soft, loose roll.

## LESSON VIII

### THE VARSITY

THE VARSITY BOB is one of the modes much sought after by younger girls. Although the sides are long, the waving shortens them and the hair is well shaped at the back, furnishing an excellent neckline.

To give the best effect to the finished bob the hair should be, when combed out perfectly straight, almost shoulder length at the sides. If it is very much shorter than this, it is not practical to try to attractively dress it with the large sleek waves so important in this particular hair style.

Slanting waves in this, as in every fashion, give it the artistic touch necessary. In dealing with the many varieties of rounded forms which exist in women's faces, heads and

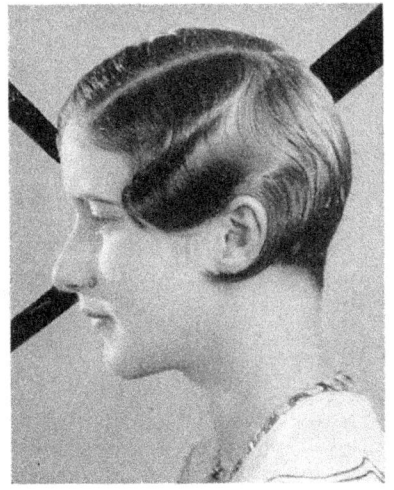

*Figure 2*

necks, the only way to secure a harmonious arrangement of the hair is through the use of waves correctly curved.

In order to make the hair lie smooth and close to the head, thin it out and shape it. To do this hold the ends of the hair in your hand, but not tightly enough to cause an unpleasant pull on the head of the patron, and with the scissors at an angle, work up and down. Cut only the hair on the underneath side of the strand so that there are no protruding ends on the top. The hair is combed back from the forehead before the tapering begins as that is the way it is finally worn, and it must therefore be combed in the same way while the cutting is being done.

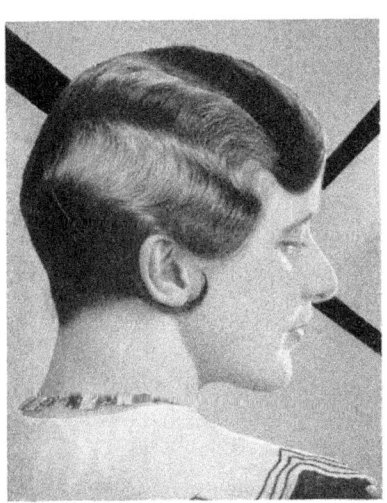

*Figure 1*

The correct neckline plays the most important part in the whole process of hair cutting, and if the hair is cut according to the shape of the head and the length of the neck, so as to give the most becoming effects, more women will have their hair cut and fewer will allow it to grow. So many hairdressers think that the rounded neckline is always the most natural one. A pointed neckline often gives a much more natural appearance, for most hair grows down to a point on the neck. Follow the natural hairline but do not accentuate the point too much in your desire to have the neck appear

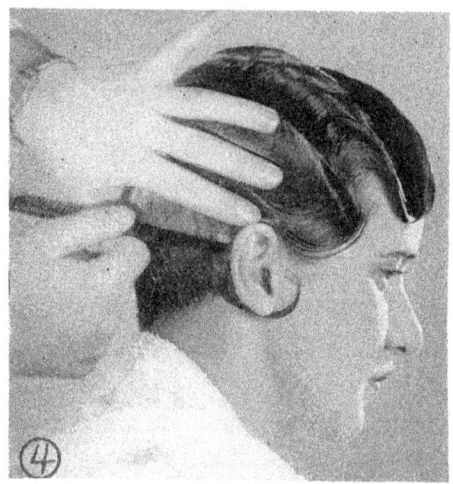

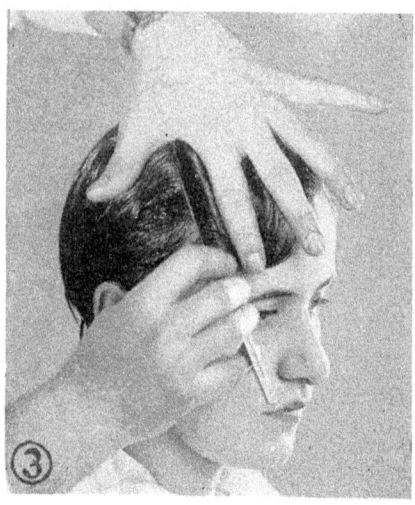

gives a much better appearance to the profile.

Figures 1 and 2 are illustrations of this bob after it has been cut and finger waved. The proper lines of the neckline and profile are indicated.

In preparing to give the finger wave, comb the hair back from the forehead on the right side and wave it diagonally, extending the ridges of the first wave back only as far as the part. Figure No. 3 shows how the ridge of the next wave is formed with the fore-

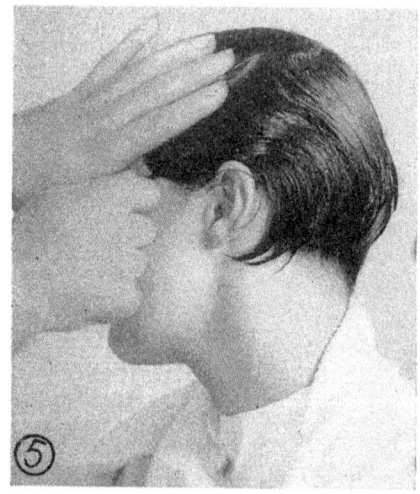

slender. If the hair will look better when finished with a rounded neckline, however, never hesitate to finish it in that way.

If the hair is quite long in the back thin it out thoroughly just as the other hair. To shorten the hair turn the ends out through the teeth of the comb and cut them off with the scissors to just the correct length. In the same way cut the ends of the neckline. The hair behind the ear is left quite long, as it finger holding the hair in one direction and the comb pushing it in another. This first dip is begun rather far down from the forehead so there would be only two dip waves on this side. Holding the last ridge of the wave firmly with the left hand, comb the remainder of the hair out smoothly with the fine end of the comb, back around the ear so that it curls up over the tip, as in *Figure No. 4*.

The ridge of the first wave on the left is made diagonally and ended at the part. The ridge is sharpened by pressing it in well between the fingers and then holding it in place against the head, smooth out the hair with the fine end of the comb and form the next ridge just as was done before. The hair on this side is also combed so that it curves around and up over the tip of the ear.

In the back very little wave is needed, although a faint shadow wave may be inserted, joining the second wave on the right with the first on the left. A much neater appearance is produced, however, in this particular style, if slight waves, rather than very pronounced ones, are made.

The finished bob has graceful waves with two dips on the right side considerably wider than the wave between them and only one dip wave on the left.

The one strand of hair at the right, which was cut shorter than the rest, ends with the first wave, and this prevents the hair which is brought around the ear from being too bulky and forming an awkward line. As the left side is the thin side of the hair, it can be left all the same length and drawn all around the ear and the ends turned up softly.

Make the waves so large and deep that by the time the head is finished the hair has been pulled up to just the right length, four inches or more shorter than it was when starting. It is easy then to see that it is necessary to have the hair almost reach to the shoulders in order to arrange this style to the best advantage. If the hair is not long enough it will not reach around the ear and will destroy the graceful line of the waves.

The hair behind the ear at the neckline, which was left quite long, not only gives a better appearance to the hairdress than if it were cut short, but also serves to hold the hair from the front in place when the two sections are combed in together.

Because the underneath layer has been thinned out there will be insufficient weight to the hair to pull the wave down to any extent. It will stay in much longer than it would ordinarily, and the bob will thus retain from one shampoo to the next that chic, "tailored" appearance in which lies its great attractiveness. By merely pushing the hair up the waves can be made to fall into place beautifully. This style will have much appeal for that well-groomed woman who can becomingly wear a hair arrangement which leaves her ears exposed and will give that air of sophisticated simplicity.

# LESSON IX

## THE FRENCH COCKTAIL BOB

A NOVEL BOB is the French Cock-Tail style that features a diagonal part of the hair. This way of parting the hair is very popular with most women as it is not only very becoming to the majority, but it often makes the head appear to have a better shape than the straight back parting.

the temple on one side of the head over to a point in front of the ear on the other. The length of the diagonal part may be whatever is desired—that is, a short two-inch part, one to the crown of the head, or it may extend all the way to the nape of the neck.

In this lesson we will explain how to dress

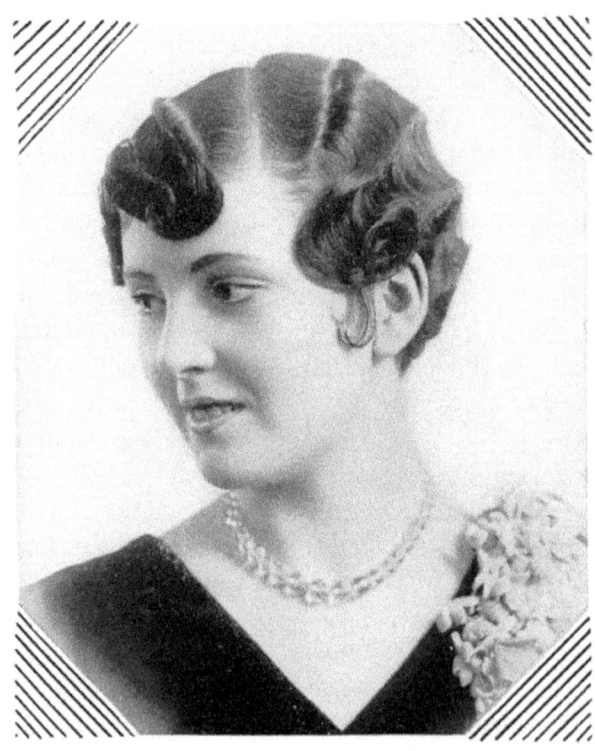

*Figure 1*

The diagonal part can also be varied by slanting it at various degrees. It may just slant slightly or a good deal, running from a long bob with a diagonal part from the temple to the crown of the head. The hair may either be parted first and the curling

# THE ART OF FINGER WAVING

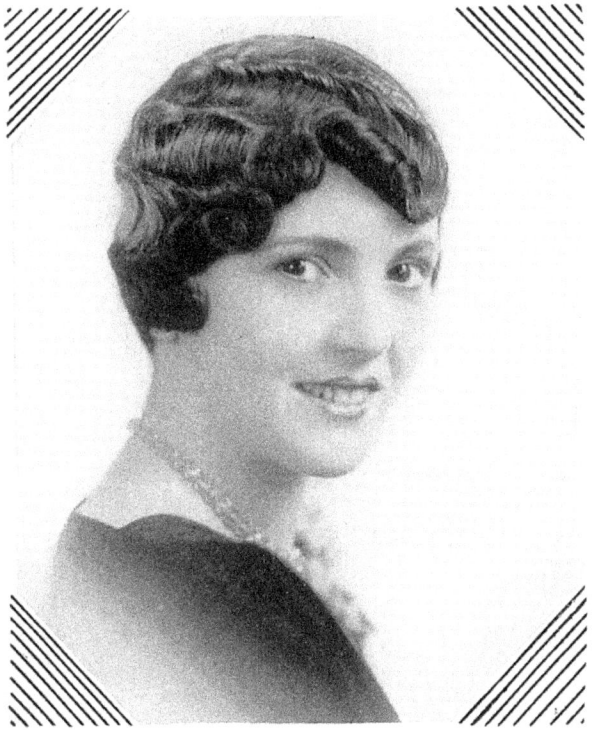

*Figure 2*

fluid then applied with the comb; or the curling fluid used and then the part inserted, whichever method is the easiest for the operator. The part is started at the temple on the left side and runs over the crown of the head to the right side.

Waving is begun on the left-hand side of the hair, or the hair at the front of the part. Place the first finger of the left hand parallel to the part and about an inch or so from it. The comb is inserted in the hair and the hair drawn towards the face, slightly pushing the hair up to make the ridge. If one uses a small narrow comb with fine teeth at one end he will have better results in waving. The end with the large teeth should be used to comb snarls out of the hair, but the fine end ought to be used in waving the hair as it gives a "patent leather" effect which is very essential to the beauty of a wave, as we have mentioned before. Only a small portion of hair should be waved at a time, say an inch or a little more, so that every hair will be placed in the ridge.

In the first ridge wave about three sections so that there will be nearly four inches waved before starting on the lower ridge of the wave. Instead of making a lower ridge on the first wave, turn the first three inches up over the finger into a curl. If you find it unhandy to turn the hair up over your finger a cold curling iron will be used to advantage. The second ridge is continued back from the curl and the next wave placed just as it

# THE ART OF FINGER WAVING

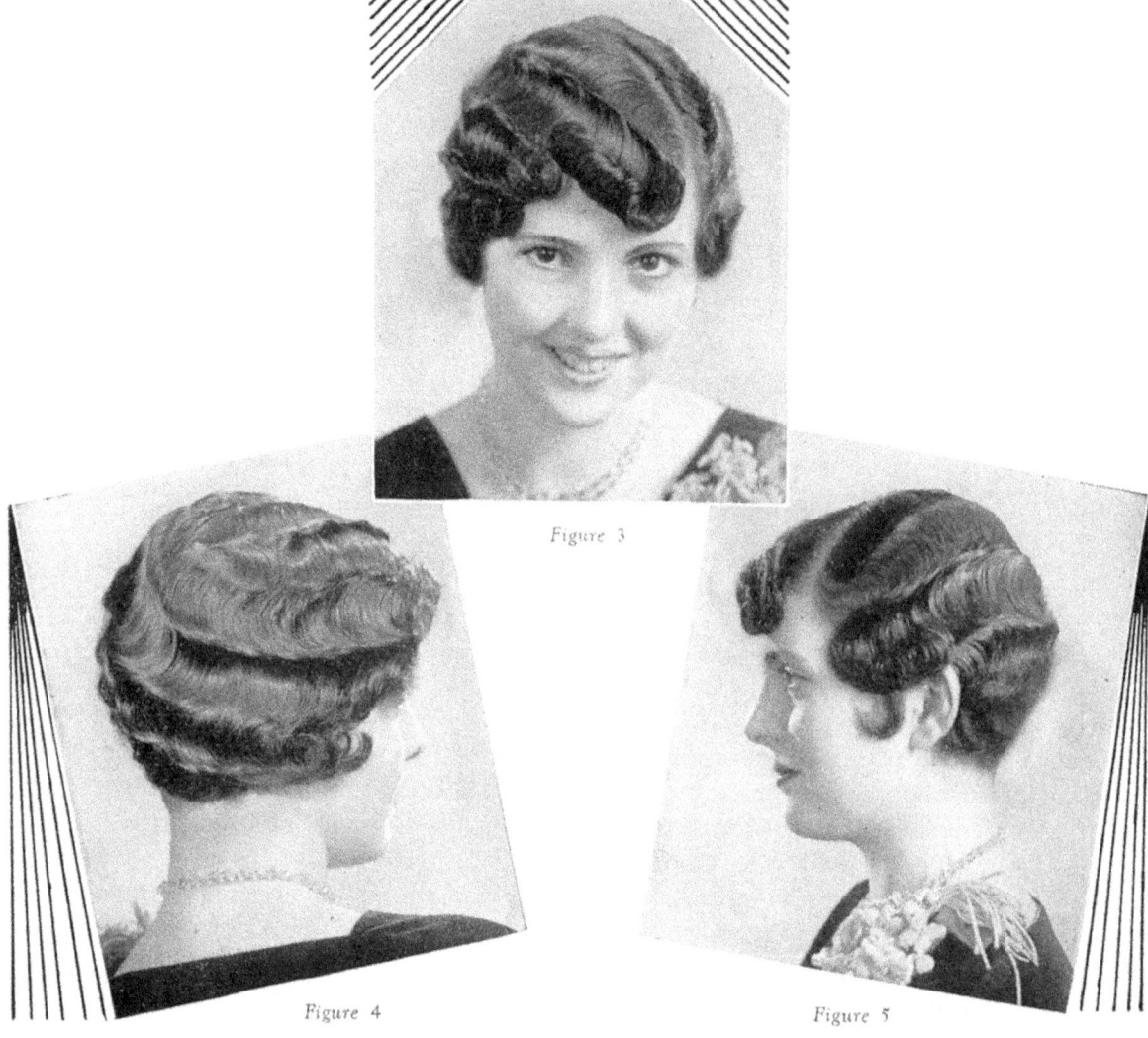

Figure 3

Figure 4

Figure 5

would be ordinarily above the eyebrow.

The next wave faces the back, and at the face a small curl is made to match the one above. You might now go back and finish the first ridge back to the crown of the head, and then complete the second one. In this way you keep the waves even, and yet you can shape them to the contour of the head, measuring the space with your eye and then determining how wide each wave should be.

The third wave comes out on the face just at the top of the ear. A very small curl is made at the face of this wave, measuring not more than an inch. The fourth and last wave finishes off the right side. The ends can either be turned up or may be curled up over the finger and pinned in place, depending on the length of the hair, and also on how curly you wish the ends of the hair to be.

The left side is waved parallel to the part. (*Figures 1 and 2* show the close-up of these sides.) First, the hair is combed straight down and the finger placed parallel to the part. The first wave is then inserted by drawing the hair towards the back of the comb, making the lower ridge of the first wave. This wave, as can be clearly seen in *Figure 5* on the opposite page, does not form a dip on the forehead but just comes to the hair line. As you work towards the back the first wave will gradually become larger so that it will follow the contour of the head. The second wave is also narrower at the face than at the back. The third wave is drawn well out on the face and over the ear. Instead of making a lower ridge on the third wave, the hair is curled up over the finger as on the right side. Behind the ear the ridge is continued as in the other waves.

A small piece of hair is drawn in front of the ear and a curl made so there will not be a vacant appearance to the one side. The two sides are then matched at the back. The lower ridge on the right side is matched with the upper ridge of the second dip wave on the left side, making a very decided swirl. The last wave on the right side is joined with the third wave on the left side that falls just over the ear. The succeeding waves on the left side are continued in the same line and run into the neck line.

You will notice that the hair at the neck line is left quite long so that it gives a graceful shape to the head and leaves no empty looking spaces between the ears and the neck line at the back. This is illustrated particularly in the back view shown in *Figure* 4.

The novelty of this arrangement of the hair, and the large, natural looking waves will make the mode popular. If the crown of the head is flat the diagonal part will have the effect of adding roundness to the head.

If the hairdresser wishes to be successful and to be known as an artist she must change from giving stereotyped bobs and use original ideas to beautify each patron's hair. Your only guide must be your creative instinct, controlled by the texture of the patron's hair, the contour of her head, her features, and other physical characteristics.

The three views of the French Cocktail bob, shown in *Figures* 3, 4, and 5, offer an excellent example of originality in designing an attractive coiffure.

# THE ART OF FINGER WAVING

## LESSON X

### THE LORELEI BOB

THE style of the LORELEI bob as it was originated by Ruth Taylor, Lorelei Lee, the star in "Gentlemen Prefer Blonds," called for a center part with large, loose finger waves, but the majority of women look better with a side part: so that variation of the bob is illustrated here. Requests for this bob are so frequent now that every hairdresser should learn how to finger wave it properly. The method is much different than the one followed in giving an ordinary finger wave, and the real charm and beauty of the style depends on the way it is shaped into waves.

Before beginning the waving, saturate the hair thoroughly with curling fluid and instead of starting at the forehead, as is usual with most bobs, make the first ridge on an angle with the center of the parting. The exact position of the first ridge is indicated in *Figure*

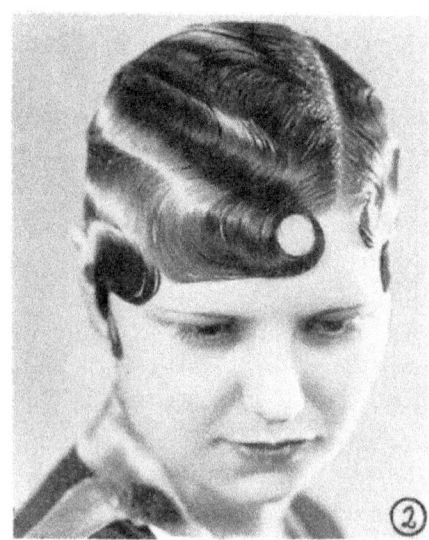

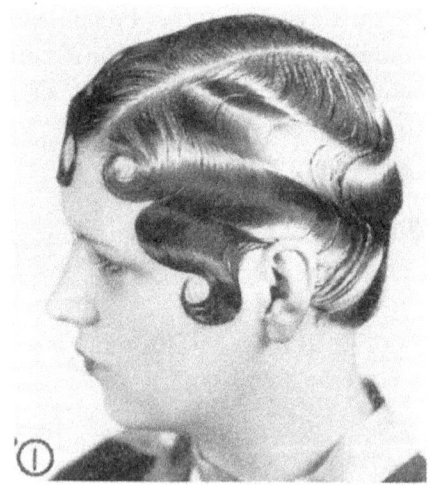

*No. 1.* Begin this ridge by placing the index finger of the left hand on a small strand of hair next to the part, about half way down the parting. Then insert the comb with the right hand and push it toward the part, making half of the first ridge. Complete this ridge by waving another small strand of hair in the same way. *Figure No. 1* shows the length as well as the correct angle for the first ridge on the top wave on the left side, which must be very deep so that the rest of the wave will stay in well.

The second ridge is inserted parallel to the first by directing the comb away from the part. This brings one to the short strands of hair over the forehead. These are waved before beginning the third ridge by combing them flat down on the forehead and placing

# THE ART OF FINGER WAVING

the index finger of the right hand firmly on the top of it, then drawing the ends to the left with the comb.

Work from the forehead and insert the third ridge, pushing the comb in the direction opposite to that used in making the second ridge. This brings the waving to the top of the ear. The left side is finished off with one more ridge in the strand in front of the ear. Notice that each ridge is completed across the side of the head (but not around the head) before starting on the next.

Begin waving the right side by inserting the comb at the center of the part, as on the left side, and drawing the comb away from the parting just opposite the first ridge made on the left side. The first ridge is continued all around the back of the head to the left ear, then the second ridge is started and inserted parallel with the first, starting at the back of the head and working up around the head to the front, where the short strand of hair over the forehead is waved just as it was on the right side.

The third ridge is made parallel with the second, working back from the face and extending it as far as necessary. Finish off the right side by inserting another ridge in front of the ear and shaping the ends up by first combing them out straight and then drawing the comb sharply across under them, thus bringing them forward. *Figure No. 2* shows what the appearance of the front of this type of Lorelei bob should be after the waves have been placed all over the head and when it is ready for drying. *Figure No. 3* shows the back of the head after the waves have been completed around the entire head. Notice that the first wave on the left side is lost, but

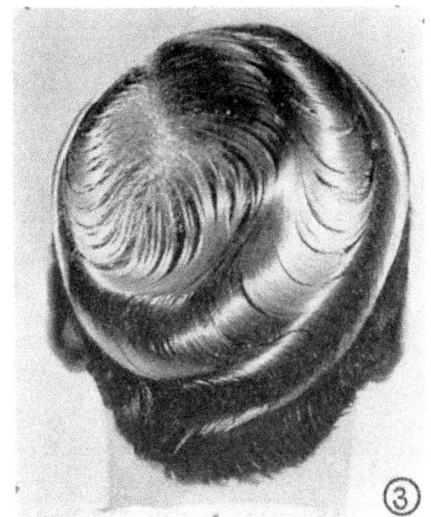

the second wave on the left is matched with the first wave that comes from the right, and, if possible, the third wave on the left is matched with the second at the back.

The secret of all good finger waving is to deepen the ridges as much as possible. When waves are inserted rapidly, and no special effort is made to bring the ridges out well, they will not stay in very long. To avoid all trouble and dissatisfaction use the following method to sharpen the ridges. This is repeated here from the lesson on the technique of the movements because it is so important in waving the Lorelei successfully:

First place the index and second fingers of the left hand over the ridge. Insert the comb as illustrated in LESSON II, pressing the ridge of hair firmly against the second finger. Then remove the comb and pinch the ridge between the first two fingers, pressing it together very tightly. This process repeated on every ridge over the entire head brings the ridge out sharply and makes your finger wave last, especially important in waving straight hair.

# THE ART OF FINGER WAVING

## LESSON XI

### THE WINDBLOWN BOB

THE DIAGONAL-PART WIND-BLOWN, a charming style which was created for the younger girl is the Windblown Bob, shown here which is varied by the use of a diagonal part and a forward fall of waves. It must be carefully dressed in order to get a smart effect, and the waves properly placed.

Before cutting the hair, it is parted and combed just as it will be worn, and then it may be tapered in graduated lengths down to the ear. The part is begun on the right side and extends diagonally back a distance of about six inches. The first ridge begins at the crown of the head and is continued until it meets the part, as shown in *Illustration No. 1*. This ridge is then carried completely around the head in circular fashion so that the ridge on the left side ends at the part about an inch in front of the ridge at the right and is not made very definite.

After this first wave has been inserted correctly, it is somewhat easier to place the others, as, of course, they run parallel to the first. *Illustration 2* shows the formation of the third wave on the right, a dip wave. After each ridge is formed, the hair should be swung around in the opposite direction to give shape to the next wave.

The remainder of the hair on the right side

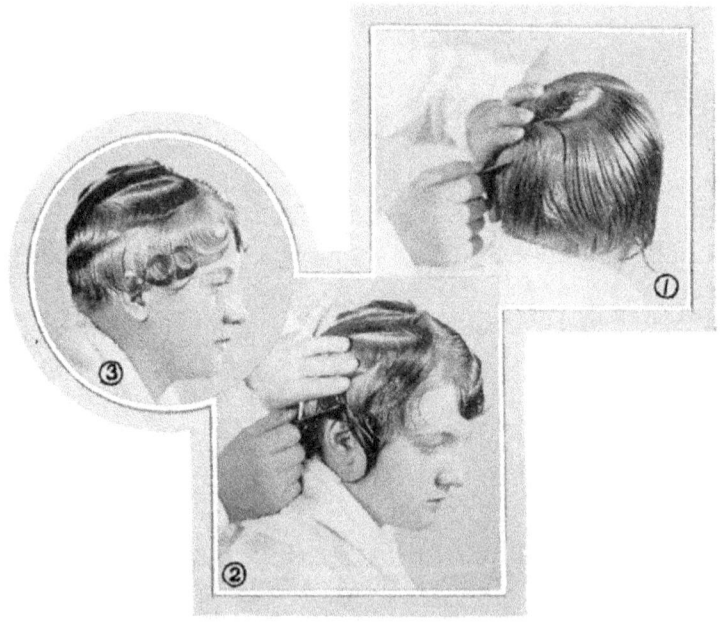

[ 32 ]

# THE ART OF FINGER WAVING

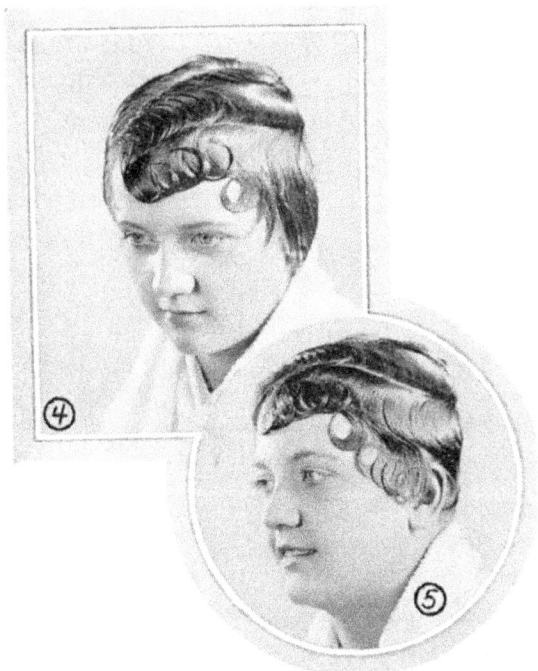

may be formed into ringlets with the fingers. The strand of hair on the forehead is left a little flatter than that at the side of the head, as shown in *Illustration* 3.

The second ridge is carried around the head and across the forehead on the left side, and the ends are curled backward, as shown in *Illustration* 4. The hair on the forehead is of a uniform length, and the ends are curled in the same direction, with the exception of the strand of hair just over the eye, which is curled in the opposite direction, as may also be seen in the illustration.

*Illustration* 5 shows the ringlets which are made around the face. Another is placed just behind the ear, so that it will cover the ear gracefully when the hair is combed out. At the back of the head there is no swirl to the waves, which run practically straight across and then slant upward toward the part at the sides of the head.

A net should be placed over the hair while it is being dried and brought down far enough over the forehead to cover every strand of hair. If the curls do not stay in place they can be pinned securely with flat hairpins. The waves may be deepened with the fingers and made as perfect as possible.

The two views of the finished hairdress *Figures* 6 *and* 7 show the sweep of the waves and the ringlet ends after they have been dried and combed out thoroughly. The hair on the forehead is combed over the finger into a continuous soft curl, while the rest of the hair is left in ringlets. The arrangement around the face is especially soft and flattering.

The windblown must almost always be varied in some way, as so few patrons can

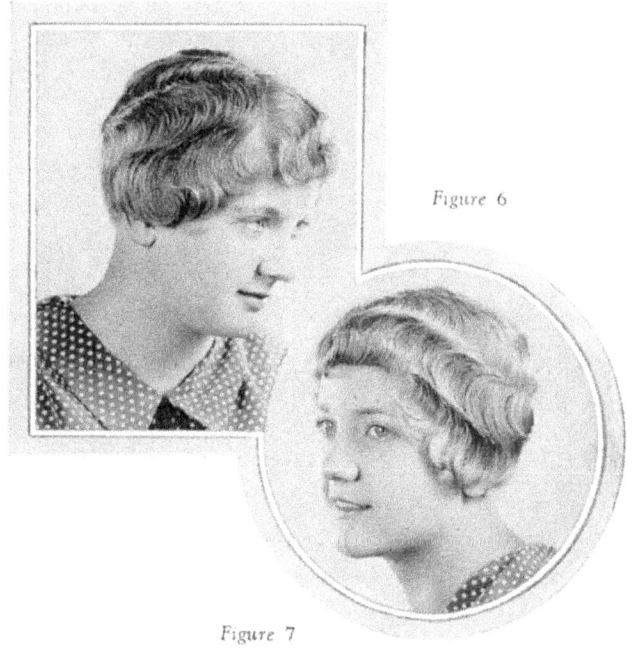

*Figure 6*

*Figure 7*

successfully wear the straight Windblown, which is a rather severe style. The circular wave and curled ends shown can be used as a variation or the hair may be worn straight with only the ends curled. When the diagonal part is employed it is best to wave the hair, preferably in just the opposite direction to that in which the part runs.

Quite an interesting number of experiments can be made by using the diagonal and short part, and they will be found quite helpful in giving the hair a smart appearance which could not be obtained in any other way. If the waves, too, are made of different widths they will not seem monotonous or unnatural. For instance, in the Windblown illustrated here the first wave on the right side could have been made a little wider, and the three waves would then have been of the same size. Instead of this, the last wave, finished off with the ringlet ends, is left wider than the others, so that a more decided sweep towards the forehead can be obtained.

On the left side, monotony of line is avoided by turning the ends of the hair on the forehead back, instead of continuing them in the same direction as the ends of the hair along the side. This treatment also adds to the Windblown effect.

To secure the best effect when the hair is dressed in this style it should be quite short so that at least the top of the ear is left exposed. However, the hair should not be made too short when it is being cut, as the manner in which it is waved lifts the hair up off the ears a good deal. Often it is necessary to give the final trim to the windblown after the wave is dried.

It is essential to adapt the windblown style to harmonize with the patron's features, because a bob of this type can always be flattering if it is properly executed. The finishing touches can do much to improve it and should therefore be carefully considered.

# THE ART OF FINGER WAVING

## LESSON XII

### THE EXTREME FRENCH SWIRL

AN EXTREME SWIRL combining the lines of Swirl No. 3 and the Billie Dove long bob (which will be explained in a later chapter) is explained in this lesson. This style is especially suited to the younger girl and especially one with blonde hair. The part, as may be seen, is worn on the right side of the head. The first inch of hair along this part is cut short, tapered well and formed into a flat curl.

The first ridge is inserted diagonally and ends at the part on the right side. The next ridge runs parallel to this and is then dropped. The third ridge on the right side is continued around the head to form the first on the left side. Another ringlet curl may be made just in front of the ear so that the line of the wave about the face will not be too severe. *Figure 1* illustrates the result of these movements on the right side of the head.

The fourth ridge on the right side is then joined with the second on the left. On the left side, it will be noticed, there are two dip waves, with a ringlet in the back facing wave between, as shown in *Figure 2*. The ends of the hair are brought forward and also formed into ringlets above the ear.

At the neckline the hair should be rather

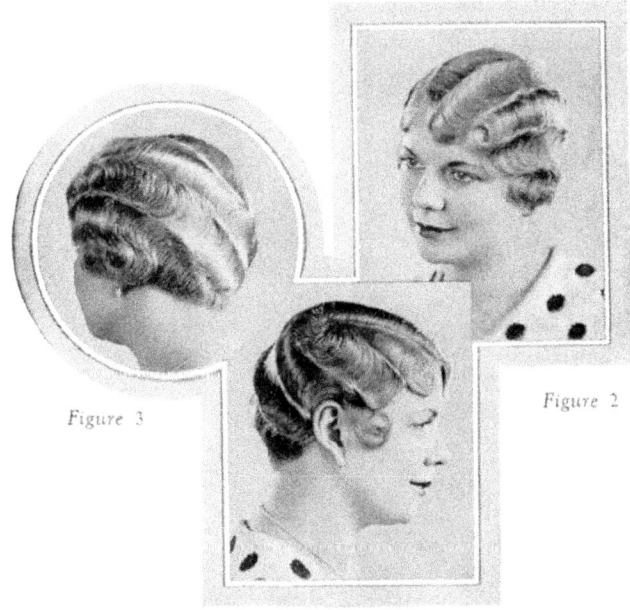

Figure 3

Figure 2

Figure 1

long, so that the wave may be carried quite far down, as shown in *Figure 3*. Behind the ear the hair should be just as long as it is in front of the ear to secure the best effect. If the hair is dressed in this way, with one ear exposed, a much more pronounced and smarter swirl can be given. When the hair is worn over the ear, the first ridge is made on less of a diagonal line and the second is not dropped, but is continued around to join the first on the other side.

A remarkable amount of difference can be made in the appearance of a bob by varying the part. This may be done either by making the part quite short or by making it diagonal, as in the windblown style described in the previous lesson. If the hair has been permanently waved with a flat wind, it is also possible to insert the waves on a diagonal and they will stay in just as long as if they were inserted in the ordinary way, and the coiffure becomes a different and original mode.

## LESSON XIII

### THE "WHOOPEE" BOB

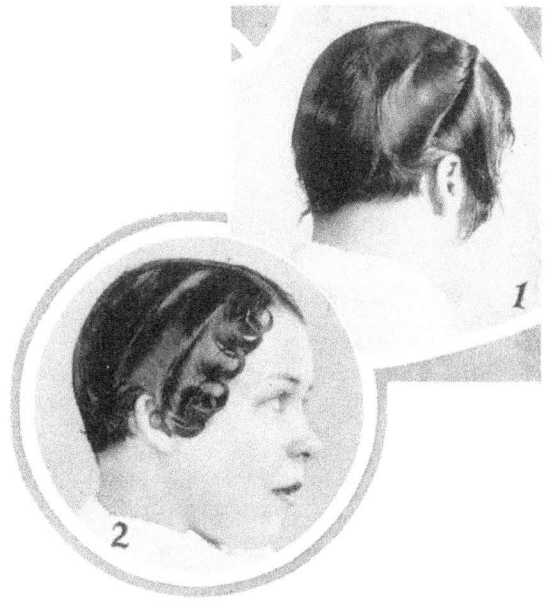

THE "WHOOPEE" BOB is an attractive version of the windblown and the Lorelei style combined. This bob will be very popular with the young girls and also the older ones who wish a practical mode for sports wear for the summer months. The sweep of the hair out on the cheeks and the soft bangs coming down on the forehead give this hairdress the air of youthfulness and nonchalance. For evening wear the ends of the hair may be laid in ringlet curls along the face to give the bob a more sophisticated air.

The hair is parted on both sides from the back of the ear to the part and then combed forward. The neck-line is shaped over the scissors in a natural line as it fits in with the unsophistication of the bob. Some women, however, will want a shaped neck-line, and if they cannot be persuaded into having a natural neck-line cut the hair-line into a semi-point. The back of the hair is then combed into a slight swirl and thinned out, strand by strand, according to the contour of the head.

The front of the hair is thinned out in the same manner as a windblown bob. Great care must be taken when tapering the hair around the ears so as to shape it well and not have any stubby ends protruding. It is also very important to thin the ends out well or the hair will not cling softly to the face. The front and the back of the hair is then combed together and if the hair seems a little long in some places, delicately taper it off, being careful not to take too much hair off at a time.

The hair is then saturated with curling fluid or a combination of curling fluid and water and the surplus fluid removed from the ends of the hair with the fine end of the comb. The waving is started on the right side back, just below the crown of the head. Press the first finger of the left hand against the head on a slant at the angle which the first wave assumes. The comb is then inserted and the hair drawn to the left and pushed up slightly to make the first ridge. Do not try to wave too much of the hair at the same time, usually an inch or two is all that can be handled at

# THE ART OF FINGER WAVING

one time. As mentioned so often before, the important thing to remember in finger waving is to insert the comb all the way to the scalp, and be sure that every hair is pressed into the wave and not just the top layer. The ridge is then continued up to the part, as shown in *Figure No. 1*. Starting at the part this time, work back to the place where the first ridge was started.

The first wave is now completed, so begin again from the place where you left off at the back and work up to the part once more. Working back and forth in this manner saves a great deal of time.

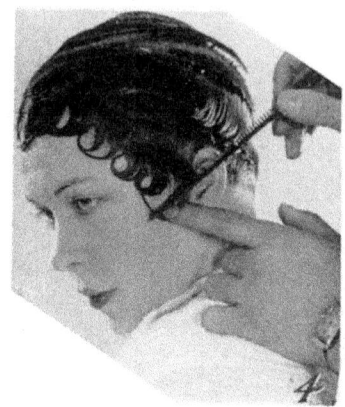

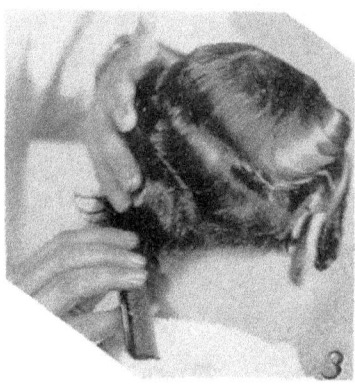

Instead of waving the hair right up to the part a small portion is combed straight and the ends curled as shown in *Figure 2*. Notice that the slant of the wave is almost vertical to the part. The ends of the hair coming out on the face are then turned up into flat curls to finish off the third wave, as is also shown in *Figure No. 2*.

After completing the right side, the lower ridge of the first wave at the back is picked up and continued around the back of the head up and around to the left side of the part, making the first ridge on the left side. This ridge should end in about the same relative position as the first ridge on the right side.

The lower ridge of the first wave on the left side is started at the part at the same place as the lower ridge of the first wave was on the right side. The ridge follows the first one around the back of the head, forming the lower ridge of the first wave in the back indicated in *Figure No. 3*.

Contrary to rule, now start at the part again to form the lower ridge of the second wave and work around to the nape of the neck, where the wave fades into the hair-line. Starting at the back where you left off the last ridge, start the fourth ridge, as shown in *Figure No. 3* and work towards the front.

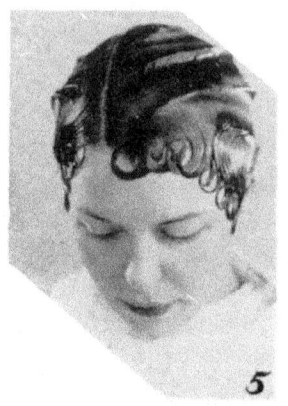

# THE ART OF FINGER WAVING

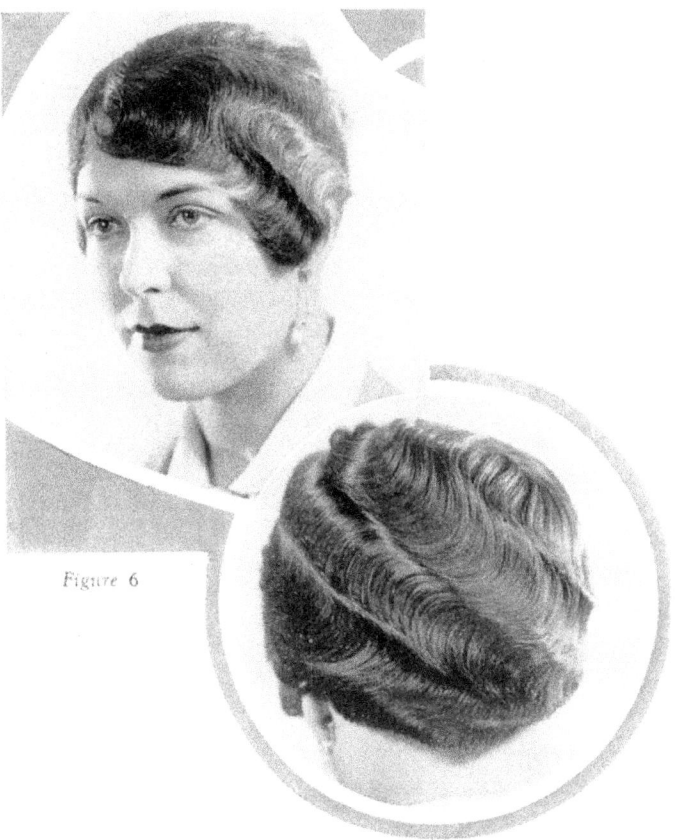

Figure 6

Figure 7

This ridge does not run all the way to the part, as can be seen in *Figure No. 4*, but stops at just about the point of the eyebrow. One more ridge is started at this point, just running back to the ear.

For one inch back on the part on the left side the hair is combed out straight and shaped into a curl. The third ridge at the front is then held between the index finger and the second finger and the hair placed as though you were going to make a ridge only instead of the ridge being made, the hair is turned and made into ringlet curls, as illustrated in *Figure No. 5*. The fifth wave is also finished off with curls at the side, as in *Figure No. 4*. If one wants to have sculptured curls on this hairdress, instead of the fringe, hold them tighter and do not blend them together when the hair is dried.

After the wave has been completed it is necessary to go all over the ridges and sharpen them if you wish a lasting wave. The ridges are sharpened by placing the ridge between the index finger and the second finger and inserting the fine end of the comb next to the index finger and pressing the ridge up against the second finger with the comb just as has been explained in previous lessons.

The wave in between the ridges should also be combed through with the fine end of the comb to give that patent leather effect which is essential to the wave. Remember always it is important to use a small comb if you wish to be an expert and a rapid waver. At first it may seem a little hard, but after you get used to it you will never go back to the large comb.

If a net is placed carefully over the ringlet curls, it will not be necessary to use hairpins to hold them in place. After the hair has been thoroughly dried, it is combed out so that it will form a very soft line around the face.

The photographs of the finished hairdress in *Figures 7 and 8* show a view of the fringe of hair which extends out around the face at the side and of the decided swirl of the hair at the back of the head.

## LESSON XIV

### THE CINCY BOB

AMONG the most charming modes for the short bob are those, which cling to the ever-popular combination of the swirl and fringe styles. Patrons who have decided against long hair and who do not care for the long bob are turning more and more to coiffures in which the hair is combed forward and arranged flatteringly around the face.

In waving bobbed hair most hairdressers find their greatest difficulty in arranging the hair at the back of the head so as to give an artistic effect. By means of the swirl and a natural neck-line, the back view of the hair-dress may be made just as attractive as the sides of this original hair style.

In dressing the bob shown here, if the hair is carefully thinned out before it is waved it will stay in place when it is combed forward and will lie so flat that the waves may be easily inserted to slant toward the front.

A few preliminary instructions are given here for the proper tapering of the hair for the Cincy Bob. When the hair is being cut, it should not be combed straight down from the part, as would ordinarily be done, but should be combed forward at the angle at which it will finally be worn. As the hair is parted on the right side, the left is the heavy side, and requires the most thinning out.

At the forehead, after a sufficient length of hair has been allowed for the insertion of one dip wave, the ends are tapered well for about an inch and one-half. The correct position of the hands and the scissors at the end of the first movement is shown in *Figure No. 1*. The hair is divided into thin strands and only a few hairs of the strand are cut by each stroke of the scissors, so that all the hair on the forehead will be of different lengths and will fall easily into soft tendrils. The scissors are always held at a slight angle, with the points tending toward the top of the strand of hair and the handles toward the ends.

After the hair has been cut to the correct length the thinning out is begun. A part is made about an inch from the original one, and this section of hair is pinned, as shown in *Figure 2*, while the next layer is being thinned out. When this layer of hair has been cut, another part may be made an inch further down, and the thinning continued. The movement, illustrated in *Figure 3*, is similar to that used in tapering the ends of the hair, but is continued further up toward the scalp. The amount of hair which is to be removed must be governed by the thickness of the hair. If the hair has a natural or a permanent wave, correct thinning out will encourage it.

On the right side the hair is thinned out in just the same way. As the part is made on a slight diagonal, the hair will need more thinning at the back on the right side and at the front on the left side. It is most essential in giving this type of hair cut to allow the hair

# THE ART OF FINGER WAVING

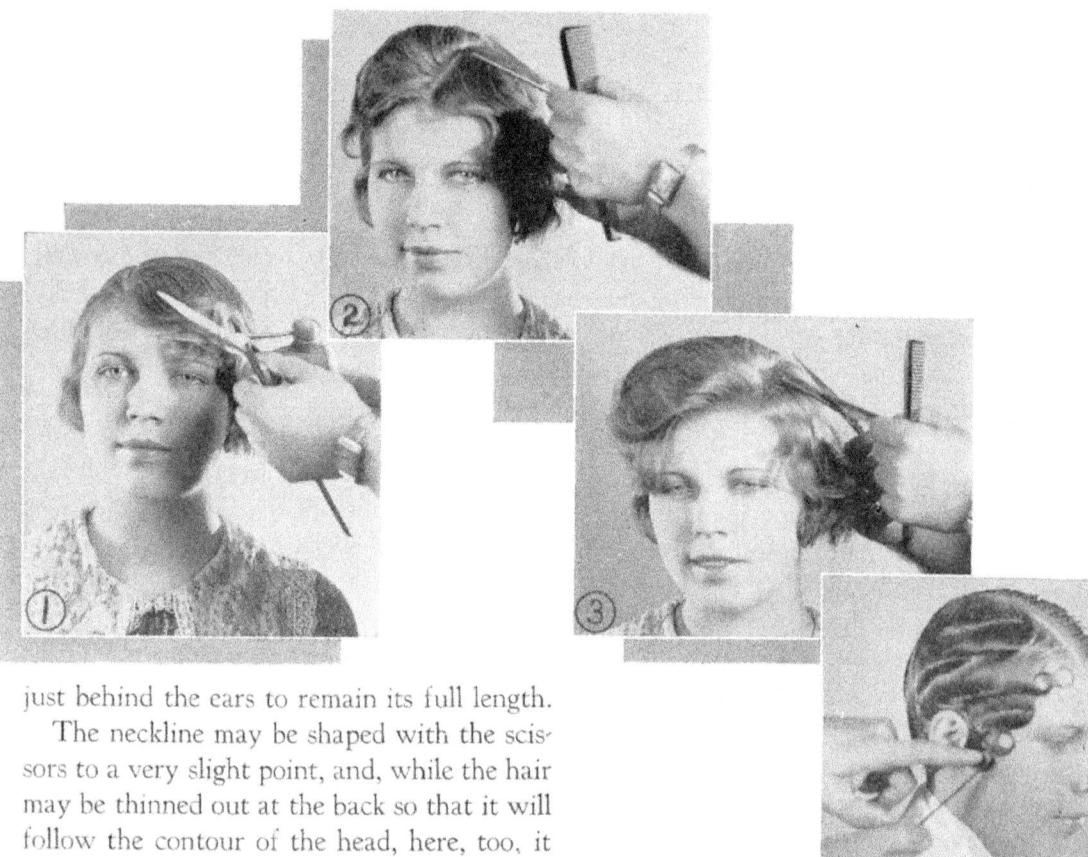

just behind the ears to remain its full length.

The neckline may be shaped with the scissors to a very slight point, and, while the hair may be thinned out at the back so that it will follow the contour of the head, here, too, it must be left as long as possible, so that the best swirl effect may be obtained.

The first ridge made is begun at the center of the part on the right side and is continued on a downward slant along the side of the head. The waves should be made wide unless the hair is quite short, in which case they will have to be narrowed so that the two dip waves can be made. The waves on the right may be completed before those on the left are begun. Two tiny ringlets are made at the forehead just next to the part, and two more ringlets are made in front of the ear, one a little higher than the other, as may be seen in *Figure No. 4*.

None of the ridges are dropped. The first is continued around to the left side, where it ends at a point just opposite that where it started, so as to form a complete circle at the top of the head. After this first ridge is inserted there can be little trouble with the others, as they are all parallel to it. The second is continued to the left side, where it forms the first ridge of the dip. The joining of the waves is clearly shown in *Figure No. 5*.

Near the neck-line, where the hair is quite fine and short, only a faint shadow wave, which is quite ridgeless, is inserted. If a ridge were made in the short back hair after the hair had been dried and combed this wave would not match the others well and would not lie flat to the head. On quite heavy hair ridges may be raised a little, but never on a head of hair of ordinary thickness.

After the dip wave has been made, three flat ringlet curls are made of the ends of the hair on the forehead, as may be seen in *Figure No. 6*. If only a very small strand of hair is taken at a time and it is lifted into place with the fingers, the ringlet will stay in much better than if a larger strand were taken and merely combed into place. The ends of the hair, just in front of the ear, are treated in the same way. Ringlets add softness to this style.

After the hair has been thoroughly dried, it should be combed carefully in the correct direction, the waves again shaped with the fingers and the ringlets combed together.

In *Figure No. 7* the slightly diagonal part may be seen and the angle at which the ridges run from this part. The ringlets on the forehead soften what would otherwise be a somewhat trying line. In the next photograph, *Figure No. 8*, it will be noticed that the dip wave is placed at the end of the part and not in the usual position at the middle of the forehead another original feature of this bob.

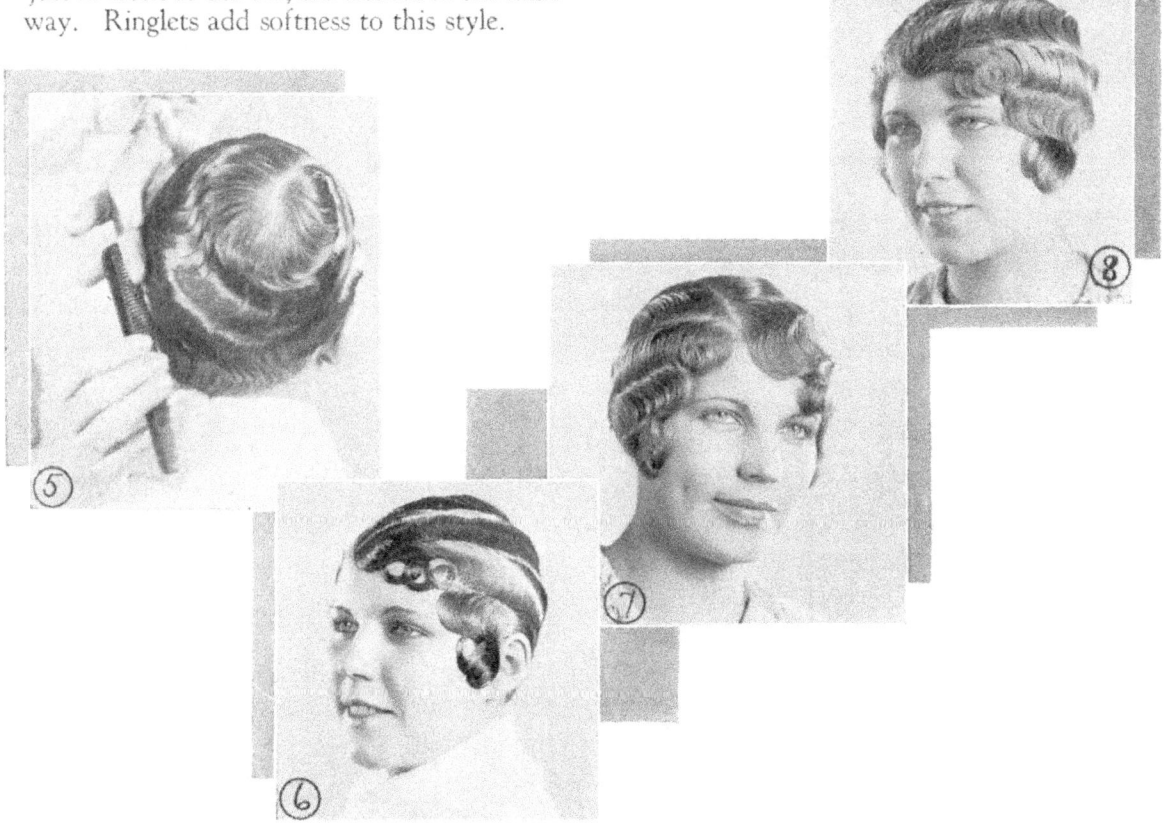

This cannot be done, however, unless the hair is then cut into short ends, as otherwise the next wave would be brought too near the eye and will appear inartistic.

This bob will be found a convenient way of dressing hair which has been cut in the windblown style while it is growing out again to the length at which bobbed hair is ordinarily worn. The curls may be made quite tight so that they take care of the ends of the hair until they have grown an inch or two longer and can be blended in with the waved portion of the hair without looking straggly. Thus the awkward growing-out stage, which many women object to, after they have a windblown bob, is avoided.

# THE ART OF FINGER WAVING

## LESSON XV

### THE LONG BOB

THE LONG BOB is becoming more and more popular each day and is especially demanded in the winter season. It can be dressed in a variety of ways to suit the individual, but the contour of the head, even in a long bob, should be kept smooth and in proper balance with the size and shape of the patron's face.

The bob illustrated here has proven to be a very popular mode with many women when it is varied in different ways. The hair should be at least two inches long at the nape of the neck to be successfully dressed in this manner. I would also advise that the patron either have a permanent wave or naturally curly hair for this style. It is rather difficult to arrange on long, straight hair.

Apply curling fluid; comb the hair all the way to the ends so as to be sure that all of the hair is dampened. Comb the hair in position and place the first finger of the left hand on the right side of the head at a slight angle with the part. *Figure No.* 8 illustrates the proper angle of the waves on the right side.

Holding the hair firmly with the fore-finger, insert the comb and draw the hair forward, forming the first ridge. This ridge is dropped at the part about an inch from the crown of the head. The secret of finger waving is the combing when placing the waves. Before making a ridge

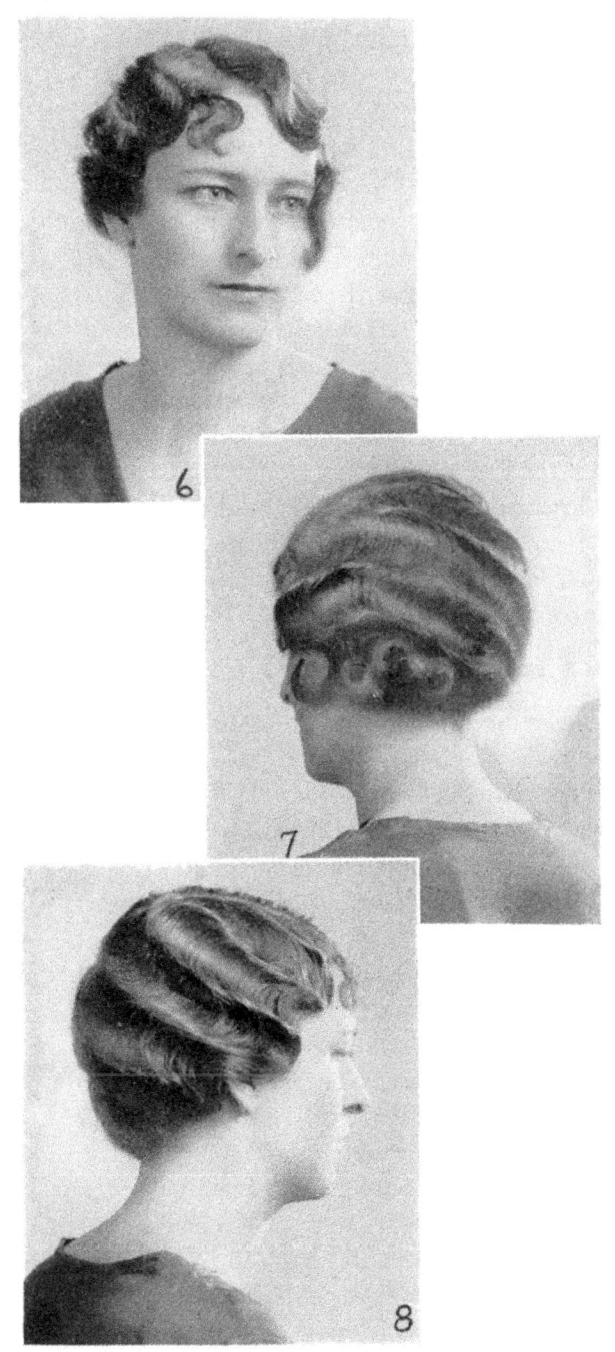

# THE ART OF FINGER WAVING

comb through the hair at least four times to make sure that every hair in that wave is in just exactly the right place. It is also very essential that you use the fine end of the comb, as this is what gives a wave a "Patent Leather" effect, as has been emphasized so many times before.

The second ridge is placed parallel to the first. The first ridge is held between the first and second finger of the left hand, the second finger being pressed firmly on the head, as was the index finger when making the first ridge. The index finger is lowered on outside of the newly made ridge and the ridge is pressed between the first and second fingers. The comb is then inserted and drawn to the left to make the lower ridge of the first wave. Remember to comb through the hair at least three times, holding the comb so that the teeth do not go into the scalp but slide along it, before making the second ridge.

The remaining ridges are made in the same way as the first and second, holding the last ridge with the second and third finger and making the new one with the comb and holding it with the index and the second finger. The second dip wave falls just above the ear, the last ridge joining with the first ridge of the left side. Complete the entire ridge of one wave before starting the next. This time the finger will not lie at a slant but parallel to the part. The comb is inserted in the hair all the way to the scalp so as to be sure that you are not just drawing the top part of the hair, and then it is drawn to the left to make the first ridge. The comb should not be lifted from the hair until you have lifted the index finger and placed it on the outside of the newly made ridge and lowered the second finger to the former place of the index finger. The ridge is tightly pinched between the two fingers and the hair is combed through. This ridge is continued to the crown of the head, where it meets the fourth ridge of the right side and joins.

Now start at the back and work forward from the fourth ridge to the right side towards the face. The first dip wave is now completed. A small strand of hair is drawn out from the next wave and formed into a curl to soften the severeness of the outline, as is indicated in *Illustration No. 6*.

The comb is again inserted in the hair at the front and the hair combed three or four times at the desired angle for the next wave. The comb is then drawn to the point where you wish the next wave to appear, and moved slightly to the left, pushing up at the same time to make the ridge. The index finger is lowered over the newly made ridge and it is pressed between the first and second fingers to sharpen it. The upper ridge of the next dip wave joins with the last ridge on the right side, as can be seen in *Illustration No. 7*.

The hair at the back is now turned up in curls. Where the hair is too short to catch with the fingers a curling iron can be of great help. Catch the ends of the hair in the prongs and roll them up. Then very carefully remove the curling iron and catch the curl underneath with a patent hairpin. Proceed to do the entire back this way, rolling in all about ten curls. The ends of the left side are also rolled up in curls and pinned.

To soften the line at the front draw a strand of hair out and make either just a curl or one wave and a curl, as illustrated here. After all of the waves are completed they must be deepened. Place the index and second fingers over the ridge and then insert the comb between the two fingers and press the ridge firmly against the second finger. Remove the comb and pinch the ridge between the first two fingers, pressing it together very tightly. This process is repeated on every ridge over the entire head, being careful at the bottom not to pull any of the curls out.

A veil is then pinned over the entire head and the hair thoroughly dried. On removing the veil comb the waves and remove pins and comb each curl separately so that it is an individual ringlet. The illustrations here show the finished hairdress with the beautiful deep waves and the soft curls on the left side. You will find that this style will be very popular with either the patron who has a long bob or for one who is letting her hair grow out and wishes to have her hair dressed in some attractive style while it is going through the in-between, awkward stage.

## LESSON XVI

### THE BILLIE DOVE BOB

THERE are so many interesting ways to dress a long bob that any hairdresser who possesses a little originality can discover all sorts of unusual styles to try out on the extra three or four inches of hair. One of the styles that is very popular with young patrons whose hair is shoulder length is one adopted by Billie Dove. As you all know, this well-known motion picture star is continually having her hair arranged in some novel way and never fails to show the very latest styles in flattering and feminine hair-dresses. Her long bob shaped into ringlets at the back and worn well off the ears will be described here.

The model who is shown here had hair longer on the sides than in the back. Previously her hair had been permanently waved and was so thick that it required forty-two curls to get in all the ends. When the photographs shown here were taken, her permanent wave was three weeks old.

The instructions for finger waving this bob are as follows:

Part the hair on the right side and then thoroughly dampen it with curling fluid. In order to get the softening effect of curled bangs on the forehead, cut off a strand of hair long enough so that when it is waved the ends will be a little above the eyebrow. Then wave it by placing the first finger of the left hand firmly against the top of the strand and direct the comb away from you. Then move the finger down to hold that wave and direct the comb toward you to finish the waving of the strand. Then draw out three strands of hair from the sidepiece just in front of the ear on the right side and cut these off to the desired length.

Form the small, flat curls shown in *Figure No. 4* by holding the strand firmly against the cheek with the first finger of the left hand and directing the ends of the strand up and around with the comb. Pin these in place with invisible hairpins so that they will dry in proper shape. You are then ready to start inserting the finger wave.

After combing the hair back from the forehead on the slant, insert the first ridge on a slant with the part, by directing the comb forward with the right hand and holding the hair close to the head with the left hand. Be careful to insert this first ridge so that it will match with the wave in the short strands on the forehead. The first wave is lost at the part and it must be slanted in order to create this style of hairdress. Remember, too, that the first ridge must be the deepest so that the rest of the wave will stay in well. The second or lower ridge of the first wave is made by pushing the comb toward the part, or in the opposite direction from that used in making the first ridge. This finishes the first wave.

Complete each ridge before going on to the

# THE ART OF FINGER WAVING

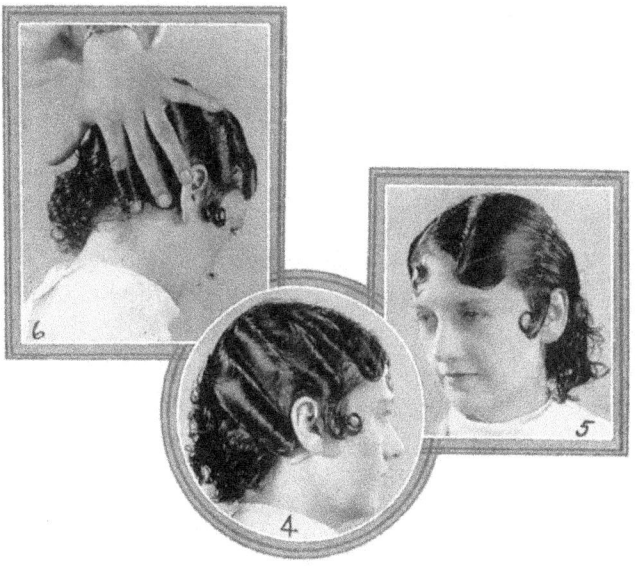

next as this saves time and makes a more perfect wave. Continue inserting waves along the right side until you come to the ear and then be careful that you draw a wave down well behind the ear, as shown in *Figure No. 4*. Unless this wave fits in well, your hairdress will not have the proper shape. The illustration shows the finished appearance of the right side when all the hair has been waved down to the portion that is to be turned into ringlets.

On the left side draw the hair well down on the forehead when inserting the first ridge next to the part. Thus the dip will have the proper shape and will stay in place nicely, which is essential to the beauty of this style. The first ridge is inserted on a slant with the part and is lost at the crown of the head as indicated in *Figure No. 5*. Continue placing the finger waves just as on the other side, also being careful to fit one wave in well behind the ear—a most important factor.

When you have finished waving the left side, match the waves across the back. To get an extreme swirl effect with this style it is necessary to match the second wave on the left side with the fourth wave on the right. Then comes the part of the hairdress which is especially interesting to those who are troubled with shaggy ends of hair along the neck-line.

Make as many curls as is necessary, according to the thickness of the hair. A method of shaping these curls is illustrated in *Figure No. 6*. Simply comb the ends over the finger, making a soft, loose curl and pin in place with a patent hairpin. Practically all the curls at the back are shaped in this way until one comes to the neck-line, where the ends are extremely short. Curl these up with a cold curling iron and pin just as the others were. This takes care of all the ends and insures their being curled up to fit in with the hairdress. There is nothing more annoying than to have several strands of straight hair hanging down the neck, and we cannot please our patrons unless we take care of the smallest details in creating modern hairdresses that suit individual types.

Deepen the waves with the fingers and the comb by bringing out the ridges better, after the waving is finished and the net has been fastened over the hair. This process continued over the entire head is an excellent way of keeping your wave shaped, if there has been any defect in it.

Pleasing results may be obtained with this method of finger waving a long bob and shaping the ends into ringlets. Such a hairdress is particularly feminine and forms such a charming frame for the face that is certain to please every woman. It is a style, too, that has been highly popularized by Billie Dove, who wears it in any number of variations either having larger clusters of curls in front of the ears or else a number of single curls across her forehead as shown on the style supplement this month.

One of the interesting features of this bob is that the hair can be worn well off the ears, as shown here, or, if the patron wishes to conceal them, the waves from the sides can be drawn over them, giving an effect more pleasing to some women.

The prevailing note in most of the styles this season seems to be the use of small flat curls in all manner of styles and variations, and any hairdresser who will make an effort to perfect his technique in creating these attractive little ringlets or soft sculpture curls can design an endless number of attractive hair styles for the long or growing out bob.

# LESSON XVII

## THE CLARA BOW BOB

AN ATTRACTIVE mode adopted by the popular motion picture star, Clara Bow, is the sophisticated hairdress described and illustrated in this lesson.

Her hair is worn off her forehead, the waves are beautifully curved all around the head, and the ends are turned up in negligent ringlets, giving an appearance of elegance and finish. Short strands of hair around the cheeks and forehead are shaped into flat curls to give a more flattering line and complete a most charming hairdress. Thus the "Clara Bow" bob harmonizes perfectly with piquant features, and, although it is essentially feminine and youthful in effect, it is appropriate for the most formal social occasion. It is also an ideal mode for the growing bob in all stages, as is the Billie Dove bob.

The model selected to illustrate this style has a delicate cameo-like face and a slender throat, so she can wear this long bob to advantage. The width of the brow shown is distinctly youthful, and the clustering curls at the back give the effect of a chignon without the bulk of the actual knot. The soft line that results is most flattering. This style should be adopted only by those women whose hair grows naturally back from the face. Otherwise the line along the forehead will not be pleasing or effective. Two views of this style are shown above.

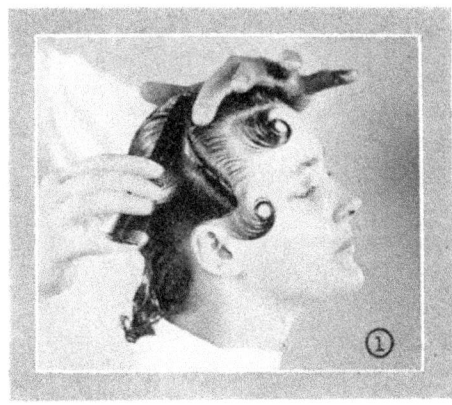

If you have mastered the pompadour finger waving lesson you will find the Clara Bow comparatively easy. The straight back type of finger wave ordinarily is the most difficult of all to give, because the ridges must be shaped very carefully so they will curve all around the head in unbroken lines. However, a little practice aids the student considerably in mastering the technique.

To begin with the first ridge is inserted as a small semi-circle over the right side of the forehead and temple. All others are formed in widening circles parallel with this first one, and as you work further back on the head they increase in size and must be matched perfectly. Any defects in execution are easily seen when the hair has been combed out, so the hairdresser who attempts to create this style must first of all be very skillful with her

# THE ART OF FINGER WAVING

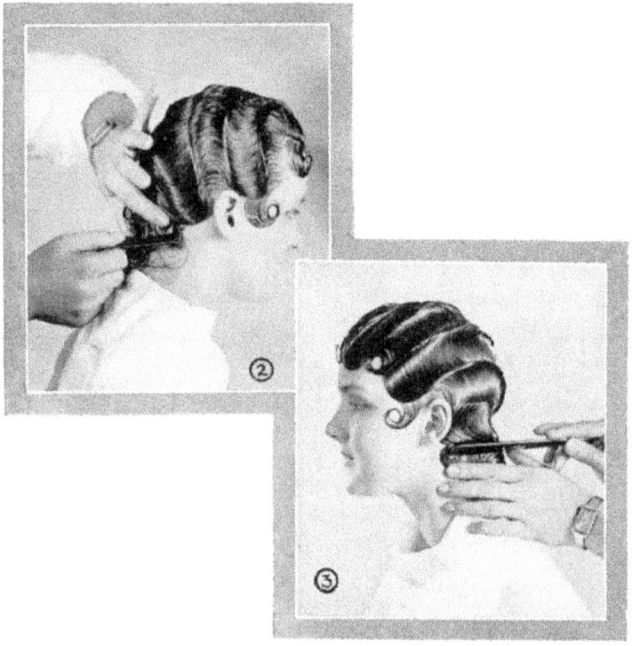

fingers so the ridges do not split and break the even continuity of the wave.

If you desire, when a patron's hair does not grow back from the face and the hair cannot, therefore, be drawn back from the forehead to correspond with the style shown here, the back arrangement can be the same and combined with a variety of different parts in the front, placed according to a patron's features.

To create this coiffure, first wet the hair thoroughly with a mixture of curling fluid and water, and then comb all the hair straight back, leaving none in front of the ears. Before starting the actual waving comb the hair back from the right side of the head around to the left with a swirl movement. Next taper off a strand of hair to about three inches in length in front of each ear and two or three more on either side of the forehead. These strands are shaped into curls with the fingers and comb and pressed flat against the forehead and temples. This softens the line at the forehead and is flattering to most people. The number and size of the curls made will, of course, depend upon the contour of the face and the features of the individual. If the patron has small features you will not want to make many or large curls.

Now, taking a small strand of hair and starting at the right temple, insert the first ridge by drawing the hair to the left and pushing it up slightly between the fingers and comb. Continue working in a semi-circle, strand by strand, and end the ridge at a point on a line with the inside end of the right eyebrow. *Figure No. 1* illustrates the forehead and temple curls and the way of beginning the first ridge.

When the first ridge is completed start the second ridge, working back from the forehead and to the right and following the curve of the first ridge, as this completes the first wave. The second wave is started at the right and continued around to the left parallel with the first, and so on back and forth, creating semi-circular waves until the entire head is encircled down to the neck-line, as shown in *Figure No. 2*.

After completing the waves, go over all the ridges, sharpening them to make a more lasting wave. This is done by placing the ridge between the index finger and the second finger and inserting the fine end of the comb next to the index finger and pressing the ridge against the second finger with the comb. If, however, a patron prefers flat undulations avoid emphasizing or sharpening the ridges so that a shadow wave will be achieved.

You will note in *Figure No. 3* how the waves are curved or shaped to fit in behind the ear. This will do away with any bulkiness at the ears when the hair is dried and combed. The hair will fall naturally behind the ear, but can be pulled out slightly over the upper part so as to give a less severe line.

To wave or curl the ends of the hair, which is just about shoulder length, take a small strand at a time, brush it over the finger in a perfectly round curl. Then slip the curl off the finger, flatten it out and pin it against the back of the head, as shown in *Figure No. 3*. All of the ends are rolled up until there is a cluster of curls pinned in this manner, as in *Figure No. 4*. A cold iron can be used for picking up the ends and rolling if you prefer this to rolling them on your finger.

Vary the width of the waves, as shown in *Figure No. 5*, so that they will appear

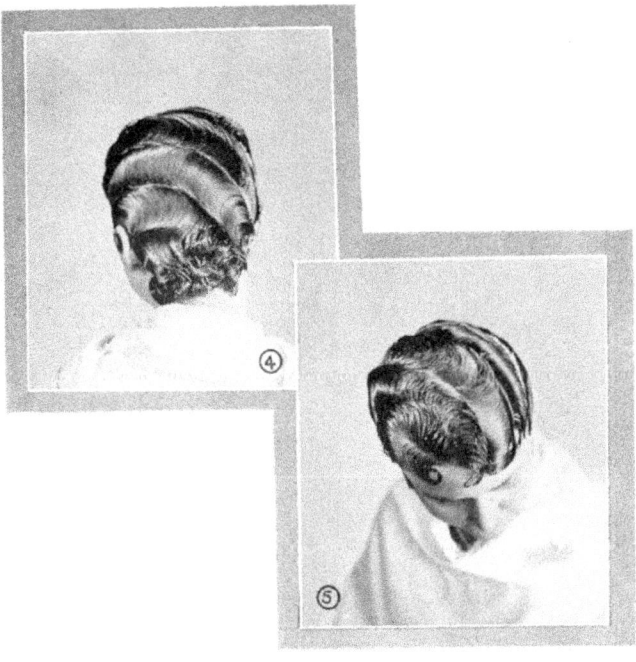

natural. Then fluff the curls at the back of the head. *Figures 6 and 7* are close-up views of the completed Clara Bow bob. Note the softness of the ridges of the waves and the gracefulness of the cluster of curls at the nape of the neck which have a casual looking arrangement which adds much to their charm —especially attractive for a growing bob.

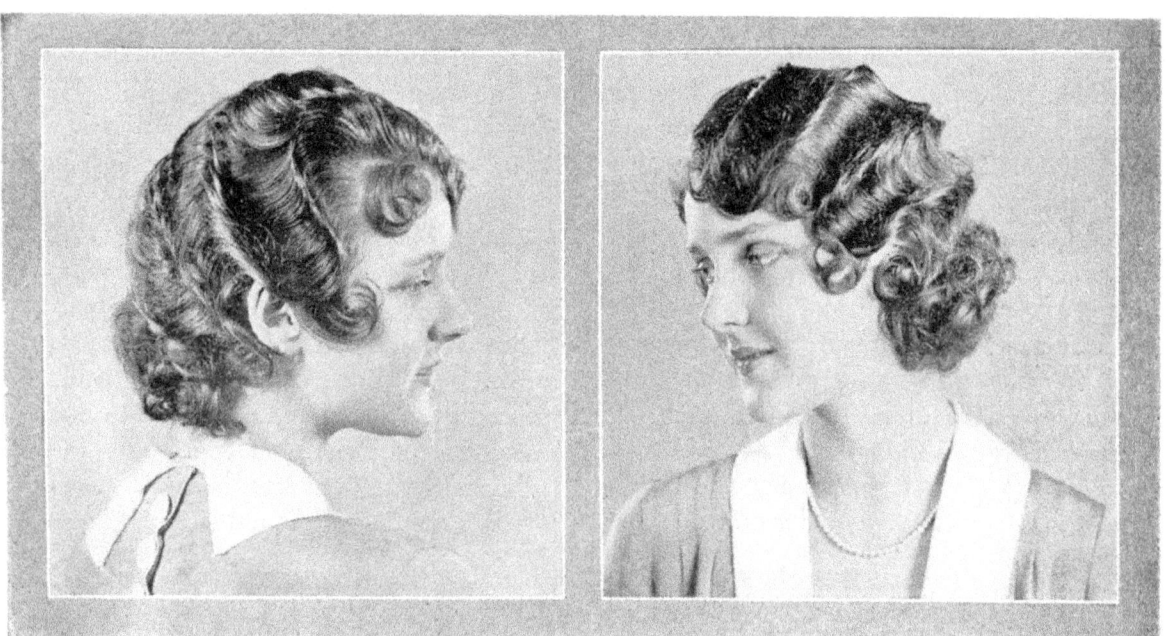

Figure 6                Figure 7

## LESSON XVIII

### THE "PUSH-UP" WAVE

THE "PUSH-UP" WAVE is a variation of finger waving which helps to encourage naturally wavy hair and gives a much softer and more artistic appearance to the permanently waved hair than any other type of wave. It differs considerably in technique, but is a wave much in demand and the expert finger waver must be familiar with the "Push-Up" Wave method.

To prepare the hair for this kind of wave give it a good shampoo and finish by saturating it with warm water. This softens the hair so that it is pliable and much easier to shape into waves than if the shampoo were finished with cold water. If a shampoo is not given just before the wave, simply saturate the hair with warm water from a spray, and if the hair is not too oily one can get good results. The main difference between the process and the regular method of finger waving is that one works from the ends of the hair up, pushing the wave in place with the fingers and comb. Splendid results can be obtained in doing this with short hair and it can be used for the long bob, although it is a little more difficult to give on longer hair.

When a "push" wave has been given, a patron gets a great deal of pleasure and satisfaction out of taking care of her wave at home. She can comb through her hair after slightly dampening it and push the wave right back into place with her fingers. When the hair has been finger waved by another method, it is always necessary to comb it carefully and exactly according to the lines in which the wave was set originally.

In giving a push wave, therefore, follow the natural lines of the woman's own wave, and all she has to do at home is simply to encourage this wave to improve the appearance of her hair. When you can give a woman a type of wave that not only pleases her when she is in your shop, but one that she can make look even better three or four days after she has received the wave, you are going to have a permanent customer who will always come back to have you dress her hair.

After the hair has been thoroughly saturated with warm water, as mentioned above, comb it back from the forehead on a slant as shown in *Figure No. 1*. In giving this kind of a wave, it is unnecessary to use curling fluid at all, and this is another point that pleases many patrons. Begin at the very ends, holding them with the left hand and push the hair up in order to locate the first wave. Then insert the comb with the right hand and direct it away from you, as illustrated in *Figure No. 2*. Move the left hand up and hold the first ridge between the last two fingers, still pushing up on the hair to locate the second wave. The comb is then

# THE ART OF FINGER WAVING

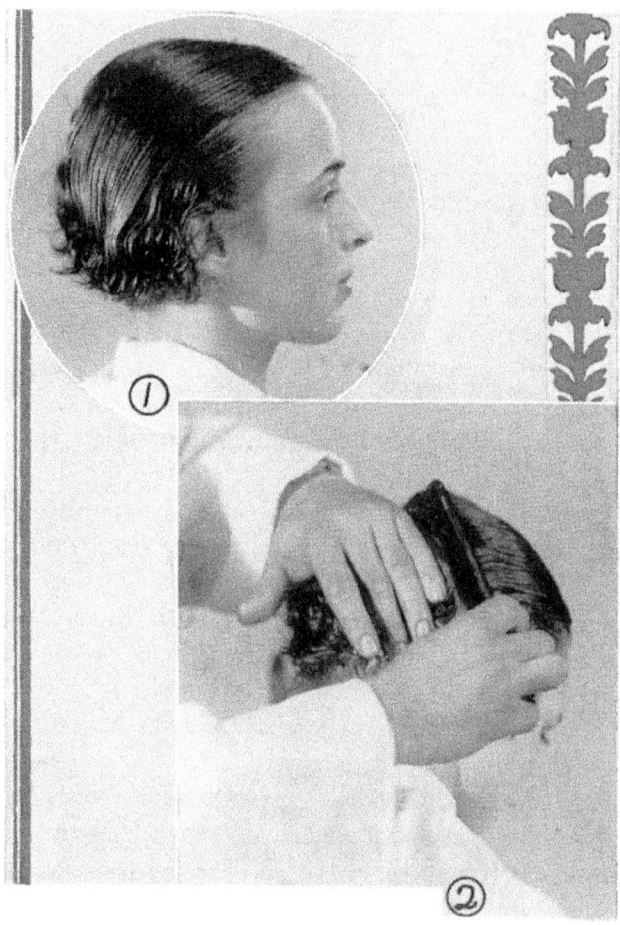

inserted again and directed opposite to the way it was moved the first time.

Continue this method right up to the top of the head, as shown in *Figure No. 3*. While making each new ridge, it is very important to hold the ridges that have already been made with the fingers just as in ordinary finger waving. Particular care is needed in placing the dip wave, which is being illustrated in *Figure No. 3*.

In making the ridges always press each one against the finger with the comb. This helps to make them very definite and lasting. *Figure No. 4* shows the finished appearance of the right side after the wave has been inserted according to the method outlined above.

In giving a wave to naturally curly hair or in setting a permanent wave the first time, comb through the right side after it has been set, allow it to spring back into place and then place the waves again. Doing this several times improves the appearance of the wave and makes it more lasting. The important thing, of course, is to be sure that you are following the natural lines of the wave. If you do not, your work will not last and certainly will not give satisfaction.

When the waves have been placed properly on the right side, curl the ends by combing them around your finger, as shown in *Figure No. 5*. If they are long enough to warrant it, they can be pinned in place with invisible hairpins. Starting at the ends, work up, setting the wave on the left side just as on the right with the finished result shown in *Figure No. 6* on the opposite page.

The hair at the back is waved in the same manner, and then the waves on the left side are matched carefully with it. The important point to keep in mind is that in this "push-up" wave you must allow for the hair from the front being drawn forward in a dip. Working from the end, it is then necessary to match the first wave on the left side with the third wave at the back. Thus when the dip is formed the waves all fall in line and match properly. When all the waves have been placed around the entire head, fasten a net

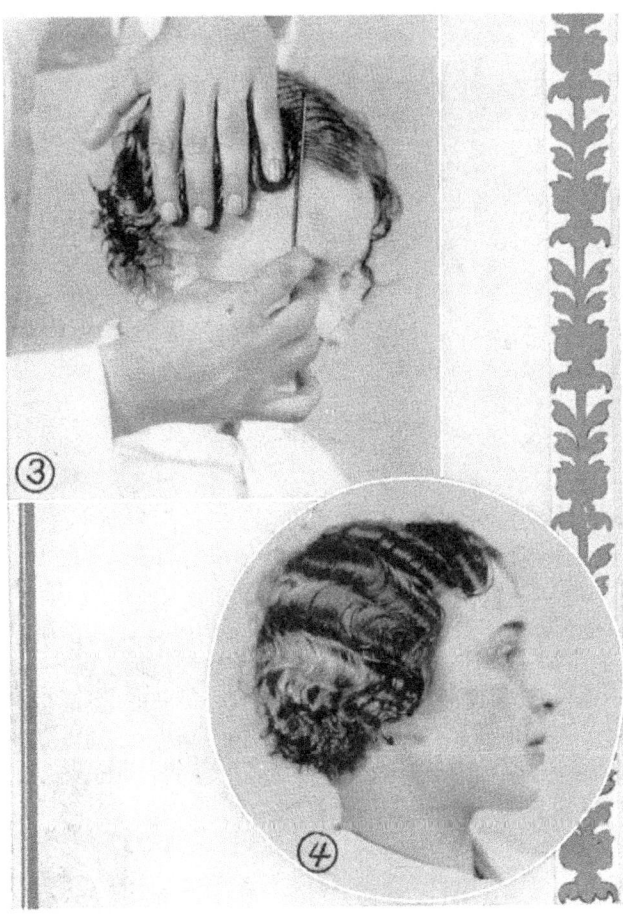

# THE ART OF FINGER WAVING

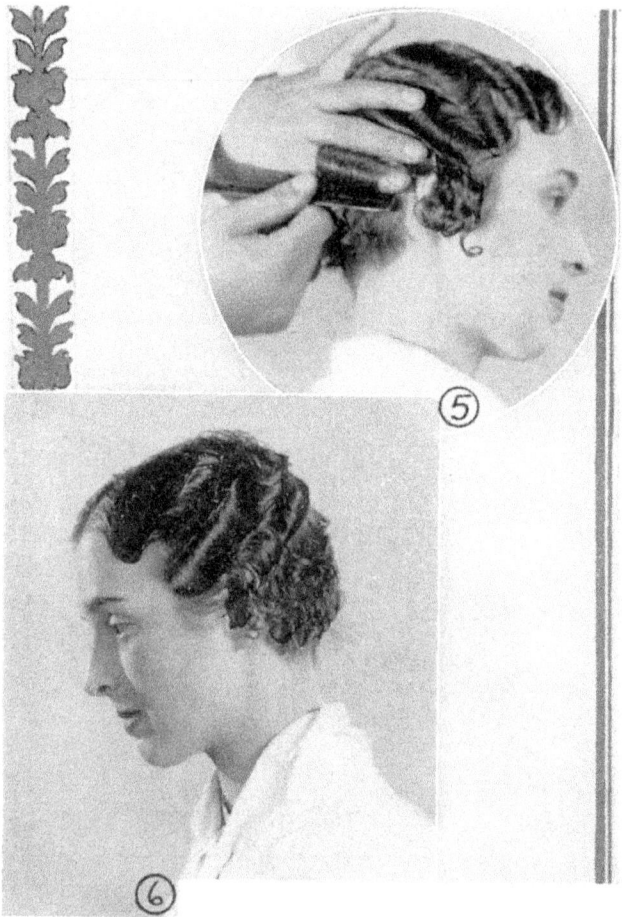

over them, and then go over every ridge, deepening them with the first fingers of each hand, as shown in *Figure No. 7*.

In *Figure No. 8* is shown the completed hairdress when all the waves have been shaped properly. Notice the loose, natural appearance of the waves. When inserted in this way, they have a great deal of elasticity, so that instead of flattening out they become deeper and deeper with constant combing. You can also see that the dips formed in this way around the face are soft and shapely.

They do not have the stiff lines of dips that are formed definitely without any reference to the natural lines of the wave. The beauty of the dips also can be improved by combing and shaping them after the hair has been slightly dampened.

The same rule about drying the hair thoroughly that applies to finger waving must also be followed after a push wave.

Particularly in rainy weather or in a climate where there is always a great deal of moisture in the air, a push wave is an ideal method of dressing the hair. Moisture only serves to deepen the wave and make it more attractive—in fact, you will find that when your patron comes back for a shampoo, the waves are still in very good condition, and, by working with them, they have been able to arrange their hair in different and interesting ways.

No woman likes to feel that if she touches her hair after she leaves the beauty shop, the wave will be ruined, so she is particularly satisfied. After a permanent wave a woman likes to have her hair set by this method because she feels that it is really her own wave, rather than a definitely placed finger wave that could be given even on straight hair.

The wave has plenty of elasticity and she will enjoy showing her friends how she can comb through it and push the wave in herself. If her hair is naturally wavy it will be equally

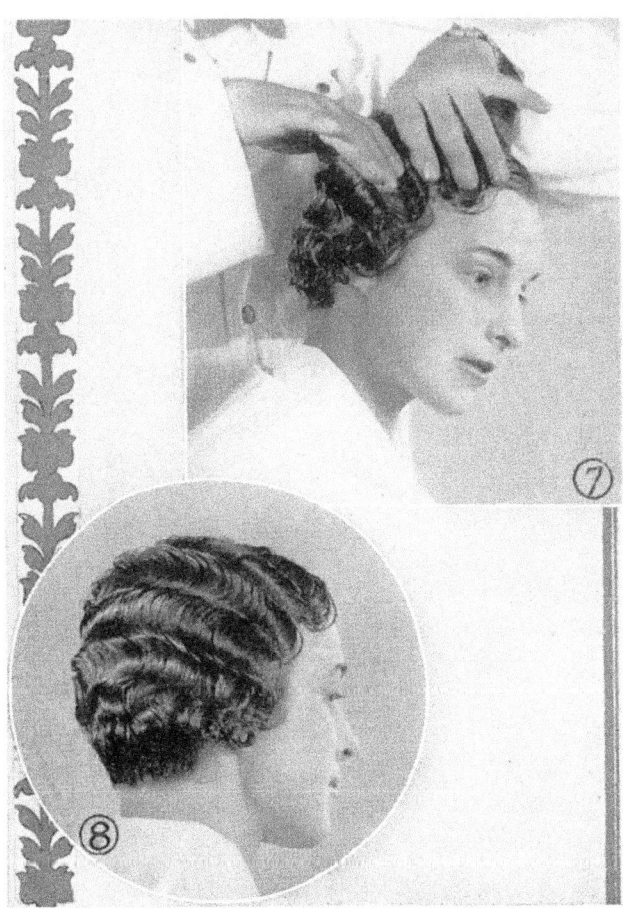

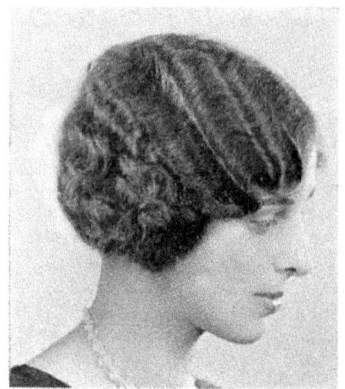

*Figure 9*

that are obtained from waving hair according to the instructions given above. The waves are pleasing and the ends can either be combed to follow the natural contour of the head or brushed over the fingers to give the effect of the ringlets so popular just now.

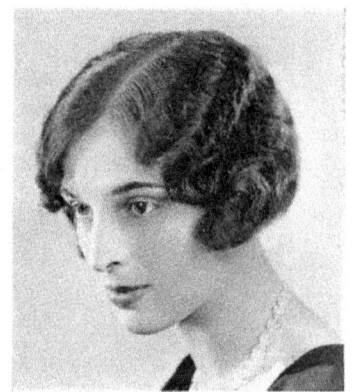

*Figure 10*

pleasing to her because she will realize that she can encourage her own waves and bring back their natural beauty. One could go on endlessly, pointing out the advantage of this "Push-Up" finger wave method.

*Figures 9 and 10* show the charming results

# FINIS

CPSIA information can be obtained
at www.ICGtesting.com
Printed in the USA
LVHW110800141121
703209LV00002B/31